Praise for Julie Devaney

"Julie Devaney's startling tale of illness and resistance is gripping, angry, sharply funny, and eye-opening. She tells what it's like to be a leaky body, to live with a debilitating embodied condition that has consequences not just in her health care but in all her personal and social relationships. Julie is by turns filled with 'terror, pain and disgust,' expected to feel guilt and shame, and yet always sustained by an extraordinarily productive anger. Her condition opens up a commitment to health care advocacy that culminates in her exciting workshop performances in *My Leaky Body*. It's a revelation to get an insight into her lived experience that is sure to find resonances in all of us."
— Margrit Shildrick, author of *Leaky Bodies and Boundaries*

"Powerful, moving, enlightening, and funny, *My Leaky Body* should be required reading for med students and all health care professionals and for anyone who has had to navigate the health care system."
— Robin Duke, actress and co-founder, *Women Fully Clothed*

"With television filled with fictional shows about life as a doctor—from *ER* to *Grey's Anatomy*—it is refreshing and insightful to see a performance about the reality of life as a patient. This intimate account blends anger and humour to reclaim the role as subject, not object. For those who think we have already achieved patient-centered care, this is a wake-up call."
— Jesse McLaren MD, Emergency Room Physician

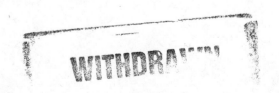

"Activist Julie Devaney uses her own experiences with colitis to criticize the health care system and the insensitivity of medical professionals as she's dragged through what she dubs 'hospital purgatory.' The conversational material rings scarily true and blends ironic humour with chilling realities. Moments of fantasy—she's visited by health care saint Tommy Douglas and opens her heart to Shania Twain—mix with concerns about having sex and the trials she suffers at the hands of caregivers and insurance companies. There is no question that Devaney is brave not only to tell her story but also to put herself onstage."

—Jon Kaplan, *NOW Magazine*

"Brave, honest, touching, and truly hilarious, *My Leaky Body* can help unite medical professionals and patients to make health care the best it can be."

—Diane Flacks, *Toronto Star*

"*My Leaky Body* is amazing and cutting edge. Julie is courageous to engage in this type of work which is testing the boundaries of traditional scientific approaches to health care research. Julie's performance work is vulnerable, touching, deep and real. It is reflective of how our current health care system can at times be. I think it is a unique approach and creates a gut impact. If you are a practitioner, policy maker or a patient, you must see her performance."

—J. Lapum, RN, PhD, University of Toronto

MY LEAKY BODY

Tales from the Gurney

Julie Devaney

GOOSE LANE

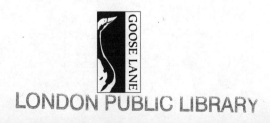

Edited by Jonathan Schmidt.
Cover and page design by Chris Tompkins.
Printed in Canada.
10 9 8 7 6 5 4 3 2 1

Library and Archives Canada Cataloguing in Publication

Devaney, Julie
My leaky body / Julie Devaney.

Issued also in an electronic format.
ISBN 978-0-86492-676-0

1. Devaney, Julie—Health.
2. Inflammatory bowel diseases—Patients—Canada—Biography.
3. Medical care—Canada. I. Title.

RC862.I53D48 2012   616.3'440092   C2012-902782-0

Goose Lane Editions acknowledges the generous support of the Canada Council
for the Arts, the Government of Canada through the Canada Book Fund (CBF),
and the Government of New Brunswick through the Department of Culture,
Tourism and Healthy Living.

Goose Lane Editions
500 Beaverbrook Court, Suite 330
Fredericton, New Brunswick
CANADA E3B 5X4
www.gooselane.com

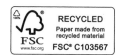

RECYCLED
Paper made from
recycled material
FSC
www.fsc.org FSC® C103567

This is a work of non-fiction. I have used pseudonyms throughout the text except for the names of historical public figures, my blood relatives, and my husband.

To the life and writing of my uncle,
Antonio DiFranco, 1948-2003

Sarai sempre nei nostri cuori—Always in our hearts

"Courage my friends; 'tis not too late to build a better world."
—Tommy Douglas, father of Canadian medicare

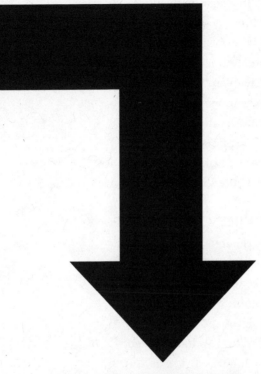

PART ONE – THE STRETCHER

PART TWO – THE TABLE

PART THREE – THE THEATRE

PART FOUR – THE RECOVERY ROOM

PART FIVE – BACK TO THE TABLE

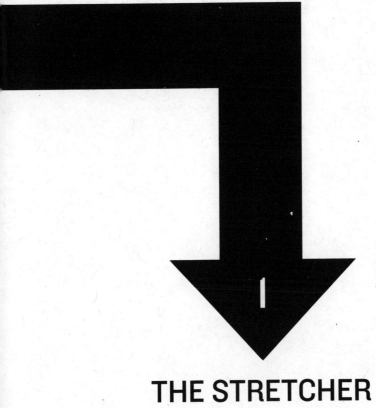

THE STRETCHER

I. *Snap!*

It occurs to me that the manufacturers of latex gloves should do something about that haunting elastic sound that happens when rubber meets flesh. The warning shot.

The Vancouver emergency room doctor is exhausted, worn to shreds. He looks at me, feels my abdomen, and says, "Your tummy is soft. What do you want me to do?"

I am strung too high on pain, undernourishment, and fear to edit the scathing tone of the words that flood out.

"Well, I'm in a great deal of pain. I've had twelve bloody bowel movements in the last sixteen hours. I came here because I thought *you* might know what to do." I unflinchingly look him clean in the eye.

"Fine." He barely suppresses an eye roll. "I'll order you some Demerol and Gravol and call the GI guys."

As he rushes off, I imagine the animated soldiers from *G.I. Joe* marching onto the ward. *GI guys?* I rack the acronym database in my brain. Gastrointestinal *guys.* Men who presumably have some opinion about my bleeding bowels.

After the doctor leaves, my partner, Blair, and I have The Talk. He puts his hand on my arm tentatively and says, "It's not fair, but you can't talk to them like that. I know how much pain you're in and how angry and upset you are, but you seem way too calm; you sound like you're giving them a lecture. You actually have to show them your pain so they believe you. And you really shouldn't have to do this, but you have to make them feel like they know more than you. They can't handle the way you speak to them; you have to let *them* think that *you* think that *they're* in charge. Because, unfortunately, they are."

I practise dramatic demonstrations of pain with mock tones of weakness and deference. "Doctor, I feel so sick. Oh, please, doctor, please, please, I'm just a little girl, please bestow your wisdom on me..."

I'm so used to toughing out pain and so afraid to show any kind of emotion or raw anger to professionals that my practice attempts are completely over the top. We laugh, and then fall asleep on the stretcher. Blair, who later denies having fallen asleep, is snoring when the nurse comes by. She and I make conversation about the fact that we live near each other and talk about our dogs.

Finally, I work up my nerve and ask her, "The way the doctor spoke to me, I really felt like he thought... he thought I wasn't sick enough to be here, that I shouldn't have come. Do you think I shouldn't be here?"

I brace myself, waiting for her to agree with him and give me a lecture about wasting hospital resources.

She leans in and says clearly and seriously, "I just tested your urine. You're metabolizing protein. That's dangerous; you were right to come in. We're just having a *really* bad night. It's not about you."

And I understand what she means, that it's not about me. I'm a health care activist who's supposed to be speaking on a panel with the president of the hospital employees union the next day, so I know how bad their working conditions have become with the massive cuts to health care. But when politics are being meted out on my body, it *is* about *me*.

She leaves, and I doze off, enjoying the physical relief provided by the meds. I'm jolted awake by a shouting match between a very angry man and a very scared woman.

"Now come with me, Mary. We know there's nothing wrong with you. Come on!"

Mary stumbles backwards through my curtain, into my bed, narrowly missing the IV pole attached to the inside of my forearm. A security guard grabs her and smiles at me.

"Sorry about that. She gets a bit worked up."

I can't help thinking that if she felt unwell enough to come, whatever her issue, she needs support of some kind. Perhaps if the hospital had more humane support staff, they wouldn't need so much security to confront and fight with people.

The security guard drags her away, and I have no idea what happens next. One of the most traumatic things about lying on the stretcher is getting to witness only a single scene in someone else's life drama, played entirely out of context with no satisfying resolution. I worry and wonder whether Mary will find a room and be admitted into some other sanctuary.

Finally the GI resident shows up. He's nice and tells me that I'll probably get admitted. And even though it's not until he finds out that I'm a graduate student that he actually makes eye contact, at least we have a conversation. He quickly stops talking and stands at attention when his superior, the bowel specialist, arrives. The specialist is gentle and respectful. He tells me quite bluntly that the hospital is full, so he wants to send me home on a higher dose of my medication and then see me at his office in a week.

In the meantime, he says, "Make sure you eat…"

As if I simply decided to abstain from all nourishment. Although it seems "counterintuitive," the resident chimes in, I should make sure to eat fibre and vegetables because they'll bulk up my stool, and the nutrients will help me get well.

The specialist chides, "You'll just get sicker if you don't eat…" and rushes off, leaving his resident to write up the orders to discharge me. We continue chatting, and I find myself feeling incredibly invested in making him understand what I'm going through—partly because we're so close in age and partly because he's explicitly there to learn, and I want to teach.

"You know," I tell him, "all my flare-ups seem to start either just before or during my period. I think it's really interesting how hormones and autoimmunity are so interrelated."

He nods dismissively and starts to walk out. Then he turns back suddenly, his head peering back around the door frame, looking as if he's just had a revelation.

"Are you sure the blood in your stool isn't just menstrual blood?"

I sigh deeply. "Yes, I'm sure. There is a difference."

It's a question I can't imagine a woman asking. I'm frustrated that this condescending question is his only response to my attempt to share a bit of my bodily experience. I thought I might have at least provoked an interesting follow-up question and possibly even a conversation. I roll over and stare at the grey wall, smelling the faint remnants of bleach on my pillowcase. I feel isolated and stuck, a whirlpool of fear brewing in my belly. I'm putting all my trust in these men to pull me out of this pain and uncertainty, and they don't even want to talk to me.

Blair was outside during this exchange, phoning home to let our roommates, Maia and Colin, know why we're not there. Maia is my best friend from high school and Colin is her partner, and also an old friend from my teenaged years. They hurry to the hospital in their van to pick us up, a little upset that we didn't wake them for a ride in the night. But I just can't stand too many people seeing me in so much pain.

We go home and I take the nutritional advice. I have a very small bowl of rice, chicken, and vegetables. Within half an hour, I'm back in the washroom in intense pain. As the food violently hits the toilet bowl, I am reminded with absolute certainty that my nutrient malabsorption was not caused by a "refusal" to eat.

I understand now that, despite the nurse's opinion, to get admitted into hospital, you need to have either a high fever, a distended abdomen, or uncontrollable vomiting. If only I'd read the "Getting Admitted" handbook. The doctors wouldn't have sent me home for another week so that my joints are so swollen I can only crawl to the bathroom fifteen times a day in searing pain, trying to force down Ensure at Blair's insistence as he watches me wither away, my hair falling out from malnutrition — covering my pillows and coming out in chunks in my hands.

I phone the gastroenterologist who sent me home from the hospital. His only insight is, "Really, colitis shouldn't be causing you this much pain." The week is unbearable. The world looks terrifying and bleak to me from my bed. I want to feel better, but I just can't see any end in sight. I question every decision I have ever made: deciding to move to Vancouver, choosing to stay for the summer, whether I really should move back to Toronto as I have now planned to do, whether I should be taking the medications they prescribe, and whether not taking medications will make me ineligible for more medical treatment when I need it. I question what I eat when I do eat and whether I should be eating when I don't. I am profoundly lonely but have no idea how to emotionally connect with anyone because I'm so busy beating myself up for being in this situation. Some part of me believes that I should know how to fix this. I have never been so vulnerable, so dependent on other people to do everything for me, including carrying me downstairs because I can't walk. I secretly hate everyone for being well and walking around and eating and continuing with their lives.

The following Saturday, we reach a crisis point. My joint pain has become unbearable and my spasming gut causes me to throw up my meds. Maia and Colin drive us back to the same ER, and Blair brings a wheelchair to the van. As he wheels me in, I make a mental note to add this to the patient handbook that I am now planning to write: *Being wheeled in gives you credibility — you may be awarded a gurney in the hall. Frighteningly low blood pressure and vomit also contribute to the speed with which you can expect attention.*

A doctor comes to see me in the waiting room and sits down next to me.

"I'm so sorry that there's nowhere else to talk to you."

She looks at my chart.

"I have a cousin with ulcerative colitis. It's a terrible disease. Oh, look at your joints, and your skin. This is a really serious flare-up; you need to be admitted."

At this point, I am so dehydrated that finding a vein to start my IV proves challenging. They send a burly male nurse who seems very angry at my uncooperative body as he pokes and stabs around and through my inflamed hands, ankles, wrists, and feet.

"My feet are swollen," I tell Nurse Stab. Then I calmly advise him, "I have colitis, I'm going to need to walk so I can get to the washroom," as he digs around the inside of my swollen ankle with what feels like a knitting-sized IV needle.

He grunts dismissively as he dabs away the blood that is leaking from his unsuccessful attempts. As he appears more and more furious with my veins' resistance to his attempted invasions, Blair gets increasingly agitated.

I am infuriated and terrified — but also scared that if I reveal my emotions to any of the health care professionals, my situation might get worse. And I need them. So I don't even point out that since I was on IV a week earlier, if they had treated me then instead of sending me home, we wouldn't be in this mess. I burrow very deeply into my brain to escape the pain and raging emotions. Here I begin the internal debate that continues in every hospitalization for the next five years: my intellect rationalizes that the state of the hospital system isn't the nurse's fault, and my heart rages back that it certainly isn't mine and *I'm* the one being ravaged by a sharp pointy object.

Nurse Stab finally gives up and rushes off to find the specialized IV nurses. Blair calls after him, "Did you learn to do that on TV?"

I'm surprised and impressed with Blair's outburst; it's so unusual for him to be so overtly rude. It doesn't actually occur to me to be angry; I'm too busy bracing myself for the next battle. I also honestly believe that this moment is worse for Blair than it is for me. It's so clearly horrifying to watch, but actually physically a million times more tolerable than a week of bowel agony. Blair's jaw is clenched, and his eyes are still focused on the nurse in the distance. He turns to me and affects his best tough-jock voice.

"The hospital would be such a great place to work if all those pesky sick people would stop coming here."

I giggle and squeeze his hand.

"Honestly, I'm okay. It's just blood."

The IV team arrives, ready to put a central IV line into my neck. One nurse approaches me while her colleagues are busying themselves preparing needles, saline bags, tubes. And, here, I first become aware of a secret skill I possess, one that will stand me in good stead for the following years of illness: I can spot someone who will find a vein on his or her first try at fifty paces. This nurse is practically glowing. I immediately feel relieved. She's petite and looks calm and assured. I look up at her.

"I don't want an IV in my neck. Can you please check my arms again?"

"Sure, of course, okay..."

She gently feels my arms and finally settles on a vein deep on the inside of my elbow, successfully starting the IV on her first try. They start me on fluids and intravenous steroids that will ultimately reduce the inflammation in my bowel and my joints. I am now lying on the gurney, IV poles at my side, pushed up against the wall of a hallway adjacent to the waiting room. The nurses repeatedly apologize as they rush by.

"Everyone's talking about you in the nurses' station; we're all trying to figure out where else to put you. We feel awful."

I can't have any pain medication because the specialist is concerned that it will slow my bowel down and cause a blockage. So now I am not even eligible for the oblivion I had enjoyed, however briefly, in my previous ER experiences. And here the worst part begins, the lowest drama, the highest torment — the *waiting*.

The highlight is the doctor who brings his class of medical students crowding around me, half-naked and curled up on the gurney.

"Do you mind showing us your *erythema nodosum?*"

The swollen purple and red bumps that are covering my legs and elbows are fascinating to the medical students. I excel at the development of extra-intestinal side effects, which also include the arthritis now plaguing my peripheral joints. But I think what fascinates and amuses them even more is my ability to pronounce Latin and articulate the features of my illness.

I point proudly to my joints, feeling a bit like Vanna White.

"In addition to the *erythema nodosum* you see here" — I wave my hand toward the swollen bits of painful flesh surfacing above my skin — "I also have very limited mobility due to a serious flare of peripheral arthritis." Smiling warmly at my audience, I direct their attention toward my legs stiffly stretched out in front of me.

They look at one another with such pleasure I imagine the doctor announcing authoritatively, "*Exhibit A speaks Latin.*"

They move along, and I realize that they are just as much a source of entertainment and distraction for me as I am an object of education for them. (When I first report this incident to friends, I sarcastically describe it as the "highlight" of the visit. But now I realize it truly is a welcome break from the medical monotony — my opportunity to perform for the youthful, aspiring doctors surrounding me.)

I'm bored and uncomfortable and trying so desperately hard to distract myself from the terror brewing within me. Blair brings me magazines and we attempt conversation, but it's really difficult. I'm so jammed up with fear and rage that I need to hold on tightly to my semblance of control. I am afraid that genuine human interaction will completely unravel me. It's one thing making small talk to strangers, but having a real conversation is impossible. Blair is exhausted and terrified but unwilling to admit either of these things, and so we sit in silence. It's approaching nightfall when they finally move me from the actual hallway to a part of the emergency ward that just feels like a giant hallway. Rows upon rows of patients lined up like wilting, limp plants waiting to be watered. I send Blair home, telling him to get some sleep, and then I am alone. A young woman with hepatitis B is across the hall from me. Her whole family is crowded around her, crying.

I mechanically lift my arm up, so a nurse can check my pulse and open my mouth so she can check my temperature.

"Do you have any idea when I might be getting a bed in a room?" I ask her when she's finished.

She looks down sympathetically. "Some people have been down here for five days. The problem is that although there are beds upstairs, there isn't enough staff to take care of seriously ill patients, so you have to stay in emerg with us so we can monitor you."

I find this deeply ironic. A week ago, I was sent home because I wasn't sick enough to be admitted to hell, and now I am too sick to get a bed and I'm stuck in hospital purgatory. I finally fall asleep. I wake up to my stretcher being moved at about two in the morning. They need my rectangle of space for someone else. I am moved into a storage space in the part of the emergency ward where people are admitted for psychiatric treatment. Restraining devices, needles, and tubing are stored on shelves all around me. The washroom is a good trek around corners and through doors. It consists of two stalls to share with the entire emergency room: patients and visitors. Not exactly ideal for a colitis patient who has frequent and urgent diarrhea.

My closet-stall is a constant bustle of activity as new patients arrive and nurses come to get more restraining devices. I decide that if I'm stuck here anyway, I might as well be entertaining. So the nurses often end up in my closet, chatting with me.

"Wow, you have colitis. That's really shitty."

I look up at the friendly male nurse with one eyebrow raised. I emphatically deadpan, "Yes, yes it is."

Immediately realizing the terrible pun, he apologizes profusely, and we both laugh.

"It's such a weird disease," he says. "Two of my friends have it. One has gone into remission and he practically lives on pizza and beer, with no flare-ups. Another does everything she's supposed to, eats well, is compliant with all her medications, and she's still getting symptoms. I have to give her iron injections because she's so anemic."

It's the best insight into autoimmunity any health care professional has given me so far. Unpredictable, different for everyone, and no one understands why. Another nurse joins us, and we realize that we recognize each other from a health care protest across the street six months earlier. This definitely scores me points. I get extra attention from the staff, who now treat me fully as their equal, and are open and honest about the state of the ward. The overcrowding has apparently been getting steadily worse, with no end in sight. They leave their cordless phone in my closet so I can use it whenever I want to.

My friend Martine from Toronto happens to be in town, so she comes to visit, spending an entire hour looking for my closet. Blair spends a lot of time in the closet with me, and my roommates come back to see me too. The steroid treatment coursing through my body intravenously is finally working, easing the pain of my joints and abdomen.

During my second day in the closet, I manage to read my chart, which is still sitting at the foot of my stretcher after they bring me back from some tests. I feel like I am in grade three, surreptitiously trying to read my report card through the sealed envelope before I get home to deliver it to my mum.

"Looks extremely ill. Friendly, seems in good spirits. Very pleasant but still feeling very sick…"

This moment provides my first insight into just how vulnerable patients are to subjective commentary that any professional can write in their chart. I get top marks for hygiene, which is exciting. My friend Ethan, who is in med school, tells me that this hospital is known in Vancouver as being the "downtown" hospital, reputedly packed out with homeless people with drug addictions. The hygiene checklist is a code: *She's clean. Not one of "them."*

This evidence of exactly how patients are being monitored keeps me constantly second-guessing myself about how I might be appearing to health care professionals. At the same time, I spend most of my days drifting off in a combination of discomfort and boredom, staring at the ceiling for what seems to be interminable amounts of time. During one of these moments, I notice myself chanting under my breath. Some people get songs stuck in their heads. I get political chants from demonstrations. This time it was one from the G8 demos in Calgary a month earlier.

"Suharto, Bin Laden, and Pinochet—all created by the CIA!"

It occurs to me that if anyone hears me muttering the names of foreign dictators and accusing the CIA of things while lying on a gurney, my status might be advanced from temporary closet-tenant of the mental health unit to committed patient. As I look at the restraints on shelves all around me, I have a sense of how very thin that line might be.

I'm thinking about this as a flood of light descends from the ceiling. I blink several times, trying to clear my eyes of the black and purple spots now floating in my field of vision. They don't go away. In fact, they start to congeal, into a sort of blob. And this blob starts to take form. First I see neatly coiffed hair and glasses. I start to make out lapels on a suit jacket and a little tie—definitely 1940s style. I'm very confused as the voice rings out.

"What on earth is going on here?"

"Uh, I'm sick."

"Well, I can see that, but what are you doing in the closet?"

"There's nowhere else for me."

"Good grief! What's been going on? Did the doctors go on strike? Are we back to private medicine? Are you too poor to pay?"

"Are you Tommy Douglas? Seriously, as in the father of Canadian medicare? Kiefer Sutherland's grandfather? Seriously?"

He outstretches what appears to be a wing and impatiently replies, "Yes. Right, right then, okay, climb on."

"Oh, my God. Is that a wing? Really? Where are we going?"

As I scramble onto his back, he replies, "To the fully funded facility of both of our dreams…"

As we bust through the ceiling of the closet, through crumbling plaster and shiny, peeling, institutional paint, we ascend from beige imprisonment into bright splashes of pinks and blues and greens. I breathe deeply, taking it all in. But even in this fantastical dream-state of pleasure and safety, my brain just won't stop.

"Nice…so what are we going to do, Tommy? We need to march on Parliament and demand that they stop privatizing health care! How did it really go down when you did it, and what now? And, wow, so Tommy, are you, like, an angel now? So when you met God, was she a socialist?"

"You ask way too many questions."

I fall with a thud back onto the starched sheets of my stretcher.

"That's what you get for rescuing a grad student!" I shout uselessly at the ceiling.

2. Bed-Blocker

Two years, three months, four days, five hours, twenty-six minutes, and fifty-four seconds later, I am in a lecture hall. A professor is standing at the front of the class as rows of students behind me take notes. He's talking about the problems that "chronic care" patients create in emergency wards. The idea is that "emergency" should be reserved for emergencies: acute care situations like car crash traumas and heart attacks—not people with chronic, ongoing health conditions coming in for treatment. He chuckles slightly and leans in, as if confiding in the class.

"Doctors refer to these patients as bed-blockers because they really shouldn't be there." He snorts appreciatively.

The room starts spinning. I wonder if I'm actually going to start vomiting. And I picture projectile barf chunks flying out of my mouth, sailing over the fifteen feet separating the professor from me, and showering him with my bed-blocking vomit.

Instead I lean over and say to the other teaching assistant, "Um, I need to, like, take a walk or something."

So I step out into the cold, grey day and breathe deeply, mentally listing all the possible emotions I might be feeling to create this massive physical response. I stop at anger. I'm furious. People don't "block" beds.

Under-resourced health care systems create situations where everyone is funnelled through the same place to receive care. Patients are put into competition with one another in moments of critical health crisis. Health care professionals are placed in entirely untenable situations where they must choose who needs them the most. Even though I'm back in grad school at this point, I'm still really, really sick. So I get out of bed to go to my own classes one day, then I teach undergraduates the next. And then back to bed. I study, read, write, talk on the phone, and watch phenomenal amounts of TV between my bed, the toilet, and the bath for the next five days. Every week. I'm still having problems with bowel blockages, so on several occasions I end up in an emergency ward, waiting for care.

I picture myself marching up to the front of the room, stripping my clothes off, putting on my hospital gown, and getting up on his lectern, shouting, "*Wanna see a bed-blocker?*"

I laugh to myself and take a deep breath. I return to the class slightly less nauseated but fully enraged. Professor Jones is actually filling in for this course. He usually teaches at the downtown university, which has an entirely different connotation than the downtown hospital in Vancouver. In Toronto, it means more prestigious and, as far as I'm concerned, more regimented. For one thing, the professor gives a multiple-choice quiz every week. He and the other teaching assistant mark these quizzes really hard. And, of course, I do get that the whole point of multiple choice is that there's one right answer, so there should be no question of how "hard" they're marked. But I like the students a lot, so instead I mark on how relevant I find the question to their education, which ultimately forces up the curve. I also mark a question right if I can see why someone who is thinking more broadly about health policy concepts would choose that answer. I don't believe in tricking people.

I had no clue how difficult it was going to be to integrate back into the wider realities of the world after being isolated in sick-land for so long. I feel so unbelievably sensitive about everything, and enraged by the fact that people who are teaching health policy seem to have absolutely no idea what the embodied experience of those policies feels like.

At one point, a student called Zahra approaches me and explains that she can't hand her assignment in on time.

"Oh, that's totally fine," I tell her. "Get it in when you can."

She looks a bit flustered at my answer.

"It's because I'm having eye surgery."

"Wow, yeah, just submit it whenever you recover. It's fine."

She really wants to give me her whole prepared speech. She sounds nervous.

"I've got this letter here, and the surgery is on Monday, and the assignment's due Tuesday, and Professor Jones says I can have until Friday."

She tries to give me the letter.

"Three days? That's ridiculous! Didn't you say you were having *eye surgery?*"

Zahra looks shocked.

"Take as long as you want, honestly. It really doesn't matter. And I'm sorry, but I just can't look at that letter. I believe you."

I have a visceral reaction to the thought of accepting a physician's word over a young woman's about her bodily experiences and when she'll feel well enough to do her schoolwork. I realize that I'm already acting confusing and weird, so I don't explain this to her. I wasn't even aware of it until this situation came up, but I feel like if I accept this piece of paper, I've potentially become complicit in someone else's medical trauma. On the one hand, I get that it might have been really stressful, hard work for her to obtain that documentation, and that other people will require it of her, but the part of me that was in hospital six weeks ago with a bowel blockage and a nasogastric tube down my throat just can't ethically participate.

So she says, "Okay, well, I'm going to try and have it in for the Friday anyway, but thanks..."

I remember my fantasy image of fully embodying my patient role at the lectern and smile. I have written hundreds of pages through my endless hospital experiences over the past two years. So why am I writing and talking and teaching about health policy and disability and chronic illness in the abstract, when all I really want to do is get my gown on and describe the Canadian health care system from the inside out? It started as a joke. An inside joke with myself. I don't want to apply to conferences to give papers anymore. I want to read from my chart, sitting on an academic table covered with a real hospital sheet and wearing my very own gown. And from this chart, I'll read the stories of clinical encounters that I wrote from my hospital bed. I laugh cheekily, and then shelve the image.

As the term progresses, I'm finding it more and more difficult to function on even the two days I commit to playing the role of Grad Student. I remember a particular scene during my first class of the day where I go to the toilet and have such searing pain around my rectum that I can't do anything but kneel with my face pressed against the inside of the toilet door until it subsides some fifteen minutes later. I am embarrassed that I'm not going to be able to walk straight afterwards, so I wait another chunk of time before returning to class. Sometimes when this happens, if no one else is in the washroom, I limp to the sink and wet toilet paper with the hottest water I can stand before returning to the stall to press it to my anus. I have no clue if there is any therapeutic benefit to this—I never tell anyone I've done it—I just know that searing my skin with very hot water is a relief compared to the pain.

I'm on a medication with a slight amount of narcotic in it that's supposed to slow my bowel down to stop diarrhea. The issue for me is that I'm super-sensitive to narcotics, and so I spend a lot of the time on this medication really woozy and occasionally having full body sweats at inconvenient moments. So I ultimately decide that not eating when I have to teach or go to class is easier than taking this drug.

And, of course, I have that classic, boring relationship that practically any woman I've ever met has with her body. The one where we feel secret pride the less we eat, a shade of glee each time our pants become too large and we have to buy a smaller size. As I get thinner and thinner, the people who love and care about me get increasingly freaked out. And the people who either don't know me or don't like me enough *not* to project their own body issues all over me get very, very excited by how "great" I look.

During the first semester of the program, we're learning about the history of hospitals and institutions where people with disabilities were locked up. I'm fascinated with the political context in which it happened, and it just makes so much sense to me. I've always felt a disconnect between the idea that we live in a democratic society, where the majority of people get together and decide what the priorities of our world should be, and the reality of how power operates in our daily lives. So in hospitals, why is it that we need to defer to the medical authority of doctors in order to be treated well? Surely, we would all prefer to enter the scenario as equals, where we can freely discuss possibilities and options, where someone else's education and practical experience are simply a resource in collaborative decision making—not a license to dictate. So how did we get here? How did we move from the place where we invited medicine people into our homes as healers and supporters to the place where we need to check ourselves in—body, mind, heart, and spirit—to their institutions to follow rules we have no say in? When did the value of a professional opinion become directly opposed to respecting the deep wisdom and knowledge that we all carry in our own bodies?

3. Mountains, Trees...

And now, the very beginning.

Blair and I have just driven from Toronto to Vancouver, where I'm starting my master's degree. I'm twenty-two, and I'm falling apart. Only I don't know I'm falling apart because I'm twenty-two and I keep expecting to get better. Diarrhea and nausea are my "new normal." They're not constant, but on more days than not, they define my physical reality. I'm still mad at Vancouver. Like, irrationally angry *at* the city itself. When I hear the weather forecast and it's better than Toronto, I react bitterly, like a jealous ex-lover. I recently found myself gloating when it rained there on Christmas. I still care for my friends who are there; it's not *them* who I want to weather the stormy greyness. It's Vancouver. The beautiful city that seduced and then betrayed me.

So, of course, the pages where I first wrote about my time there are stained with rage and tears. There was no joy the first time I wrote this chapter ten years ago. At the time, I had a yellow notebook with the university emblem on the front. At the beginning of the notebook, I wrote the words of scolding academics. In the back, I described the raging rectal pain I experienced while they spoke.

But before the pain and horror of the relationship breakdown, let's examine the seduction.

I have snapshots of pretty images scattered throughout my memories of living in Vancouver.

Snapshot One: we arrive at the apartment, sight unseen, after driving across the country: Blair; my dog, Susie; and I in the U-Haul, and my best friend, Maia; her partner, Colin; and their cat, Tiggy, in their minivan. My friend Adrian tirelessly searched for us and, just days earlier, finally found this two-storey, two-bedroom little place near the beach.

Maia and I are completely exhausted and just the sight of the overpacked U-Haul and van is making our heads spin. I turn to her.

"Let's walk Susie down to the water before we unpack."

Maia looks guiltily at the guys, who are already unpacking.

Colin and Blair wave us on. "Go. It's fine!"

They're both the kind of guys to actually mean it, not just say it at the time and then sulk later because they were left doing the work. So we walk down to the beach; it's a beautiful sunny evening, and Susie is thrilled with all the new smells. We see the outdoor salt-water swimming pool, the mountains in the backdrop. Looking in the little shops, we pick up a sunflower plant, crackers, and cheese. Feeling re-energized, we return to our new home and open a bottle of wine.

We all sit on various boxes and packing crates, eating and drinking and appreciating our new city.

Snapshot Two: thousands of people are marching across the Burrard Street Bridge. It's two months after US and Canadian troops went to Afghanistan, and we're protesting the war. Vancouver hasn't seen a march this big since the anti-nuclear marches in the 1980s. The sun is shining brightly on this crisp November day, and as I stand along the side of the bridge directing the crowd with the other organizers, a group of students from my program at school call out my name. They're carrying a banner and smiling and waving. I wave back happily.

Snapshot Three: it's springtime and it's my birthday. My friend Mali lives on campus, and she has set up a sushi picnic for me and our friend

Adrian. We argue about the season finale of the sixth season of *Buffy the Vampire Slayer*. I love the episode, especially the part where Buffy tells her sister, Dawn, that she doesn't want to protect her from the world; she wants to show it to her. Mali hates it and thinks it's sentimental, individualist bullshit. We both love arguing the politics of *Buffy*. The weather's warm; the sushi's yummy; the view is almost absurd in its mountainous, spectacular glory.

Snapshot Four: I'm on the beach with Bobbie, my childhood friend from Manchester, and my dog, Susie. By miraculous coincidence, Bobbie and her partner have decided to spend the year travelling Canada and, without any prior knowledge of our plans, arrived in Vancouver three days after we did. My fourteen-year-old schnauzer, who vets claimed was close to her end three years before, is running up to the waves, snatching up large branches and playing with such glee that many people ask how old our little puppy is. The crisp, gorgeous smell of the beach in late evening matches the rays of sunshine beaming across the water onto Bobbie and me as we reminisce and peacefully walk.

I've always been a juggler of many balls. There were times in high school where, between classes, after-school activities, and part-time jobs and babysitting, I had an entire week of twelve-hour days. In university too: lots of part-time jobs, lots of activist campaigns, full course load. At the same time, despite being pretty well-organized, I've never been a particularly hard worker. I've always spent more time strategizing about how to do something efficiently than I have in the hard slog of labour. Like, when I watch Blair doing something, he tackles the task with a vengeance. He's fully concentrated, unrelenting, practically un-distractible, whether he wants to do it or not. Just gets "stuck in," as my dad would say. I thrive on distraction and multiple activities at once, and when I don't feel like doing something, I do something else until I do feel like it. When I am well, I can be committed, passionately dependable, decent with deadlines, but always, in my own head, kind of a slacker.

The summer before we moved to Vancouver, the professor whom I wanted to work with on my thesis about the history of health care movements emails me and asks me to be her research assistant. The subject matter of the particular project doesn't exactly fit my research, but I'm familiar with her other work around health care that does. We'll call her Mitzi because it's far enough from her actual name to be random but absurd enough to make me smile. A tool I've put in my chest for dealing with traumatic incidents is to have an inside joke with myself, and secretly calling her Mitzi helps. I already have some other jobs set up. One is a research job I've brought with me from Toronto. The other is social activist–type work that barely covers my rent. Mitzi is offering to pay me a lot more than the other jobs, so I'm thrilled by this new income opportunity as well as the chance to work closely with an academic whose books and articles I studied during my undergrad degree.

As the semester begins, my plate is full. I'm excited about all these things that are happening and that I'll be working on. My program has its orientation, and as we students gather in the small building, introducing ourselves, the department head comes in and talks to us.

"We had hundreds of applications," she tells us, looking meaningfully around the room, "and we only chose seven of you."

The implication chills me. I thought I was entering a small, progressive program where we'd all engage in a supportive sort of solidarity. But here she is, setting a tone of competition and elitism on the very first day. When we meet privately, she pressures me to switch from the part-time status I've chosen to full-time. I explain that I have quite a few different things happening while I'm in Vancouver, including the research assistantship with her colleague. What I don't say is that there's no way I can afford full-time tuition anyway. I feel uncomfortable, out of my element, already scared that I've made a mistake in coming here.

Bobbie and her partner have chosen this day to accompany me to the campus and look around. They meet me outside my department's building.

It's still hot in early September, and we climb down through rocks and trees to the beach. It turns out to be a nude beach, which I don't remember knowing prior to climbing down. It's pretty deserted. The only person we notice is an old guy wearing nothing but a fanny-pack who is selling pot. We strip down to our underwear and run into the cold, cold waves, then dry off in the sunshine. The first few days Bobbie and her partner are in Vancouver, they stay at our place. When the neighbours see a constant stream of six people, plus a cat and a dog, coming in and out of the small apartment, they're a bit shocked but mostly amused, asking repeatedly, "*How* many of you are living in there?"

When I go to meet Mitzi a few days later, I'm open and honest about who I am and the kind of work I do.

"I don't mean to mother you," she says, "but you can't be an activist and an academic; you're going to have to choose."

I want to say, *It's a really good thing you're not trying to mother me, considering I don't even let my mother "mother" me; you really wouldn't get very far.* But I don't. She goes on to criticize her last research assistant. I don't like this at all, just on principle—it's a bad precedent for an employer to open discussions of her expectations by bashing her last employee. But part of me can't help making desperate mental notes not to commit the same incursions as my predecessor. What doesn't occur to me but possibly should is that Mitzi clearly has expectations of her underlings that she (a) doesn't clearly express and (b) harshly judges us for not meeting. Over the course of the next few meetings, she interrogates every aspect of my life, frequently asking how the living situation with "two couples" is going, clearly believing such an arrangement is doomed to fail. She knows when I miss class because she just happens to be discussing my attendance rates with my other profs.

In the midst of this already unpleasant situation is a terrible confluence of events. I can't actually find any of the material she wants. This has never happened before. I've always had magical powers with research. The thing

I need always falls into my lap exactly when I need it. The book will open to the page with the perfect quote; the library will have the book I need sitting right in front of me as I walk in. Friends found the swiftness of my essay production really irritating, but no one could deny that the end product was almost always fine. But she's asking me to find really specific material in really old periodicals that's just not there.

4.... Bowel Disease

At the same time, in addition to the chronic diarrhea and nausea, shortly after arriving in Vancouver, I get a nasty cold that quickly turns into a chest infection. I'm trying to get my life back in order with school and work when I get the worst menstrual period I've ever had. I'm immobilized by pain for five days with what I later recognize as my first major bowel flare-up.

There's a walk-in clinic at the end of my street. I reluctantly go in. First, I tell the doctor about the chest infection that won't go away. He prescribes antibiotics.

"Also," I say, "I just had the worst bowel pain I've ever had during my period."

He looks up over his glasses.

"Like," I continue, "I couldn't even move. And so much diarrhea. It went on for days. I've been having issues like this on and off for the last couple of months."

He looks judgmentally at my body, scanning me up and down.

"You would have lost weight if anything was *really* wrong," he says.

He doesn't actually *ask* me if I've lost weight, just assumes based on the flesh he sees curving over my bones and muscles that nothing serious could be wrong with my digestive system. I feel so shamed by his absolute dismissal that I don't persist. I take my new prescription for my chest infection and leave.

"You should get the flu shot," Mitzi insists when I vaguely say I think I had the flu. "My son and I got the flu shot. We used to get the flu all the time. Now we never get it."

"Have you gotten your flu shot yet?" she accusingly asks me at each subsequent meeting.

"Do you have mono?" the director of my department asks me. "My daughter has mono," she confides. "It's terrible, just when you think it's gone, always coming back…"

It is a person's basic right to maintain confidentiality about our own medical conditions. It should simply be enough that someone states that we've been ill, without having to reveal the symptoms. Especially when they include things like terrifyingly painful rectal cramping and bloody diarrhea. But this basic control over information about my body is constantly challenged—it just doesn't seem to apply to graduate students. At the same time, the department is central to an important interdisciplinary project that explores issues of illness and disability. Clearly significant theoretical issues, but quite unseemly when they present themselves in your office in the form of a graduate student. If my body is indeed a battleground, then my department and I are on opposite sides of the barricades.

5. Things Fall Apart

On the world stage, meanwhile, a war is starting.

On September 11, 2001, we wake up in Vancouver — three hours behind New York — about an hour after the second plane has hit. I sit on the couch, thinking, *Oh, my God, imagine if I knew people there.* With a sickening shock, I remember that my parents are visiting my dad's cousins, the Irish-American Devaneys, in New York. Two days earlier, before they left, my mum phoned me from their house in Toronto with the number where they'd be.

Rolling my eyes, I said, "Mum, I'm in Vancouver. Why would I need to call you the four days you're in New York?"

I vaguely considered just pretending to write the number down as she gave it to me but found a pen at the last minute and scrawled it down.

Now, on the morning of the attacks on the World Trade Center, I can't decide whether to dial it. Maybe these will be the last few minutes that I can imagine my parents are okay. Better than knowing for sure that they're not. I steel myself and phone, finding them in Long Island, safe but shaken. They were at the towers the morning before. Relieved, I decide to take Susie for a walk. I'm amazed because no one seems to be reacting. People are just getting on with their mornings. I can't calm down. I finished the last year of my political science degree a few months before moving to Vancouver. Just that spring, I saw a film in my international relations course that showed the room in the US military facility where the "nuclear button" is housed. I have a really bad memory for films sometimes. Especially ones I see in class. So I can't remember any of the context or descriptions of safeguards. The only frame I recall is some bored-looking dude sitting next to a button that has the power to blow up the world. As I walk past the happy, laughing people sharing breakfast and coffees on patios all the way down to the beach, I'm waiting for the end of the world. Of course, I don't tell anyone that I really believe this. I make exaggerated mocking references to this anxiety over the coming weeks and get on with things.

Bombs start dropping in Afghanistan, and having always been active in anti-war campaigns, I get involved in organizing. One of my professors, Tara, becomes the target of a vile international hate campaign for speaking out. Friends of mine are in the forefront of organizing a public defence. My friend Mali asks me to organize the security for her first public appearance. Because I've done feminist community-type security before, I happily agree. I arrive at the meeting early to give the team of community volunteers some training and present the basic plan. When the meeting overflows and Tara decides to address the crowd gathered outside, I end up, as security organizer, standing at her side on TV news and in the paper. It's hard to describe how random this feels at the time—I can't imagine not supporting Tara and Mali at this meeting. To me, it feels like I've barely done anything, and yet, there I am, in the press, holding a megaphone.

Mitzi clearly does not approve. She later implies to the department head that the reason my schooling and employment are not in order is because I'm too busy being an activist. I wish. When the October bowel flare-up comes on, I'm in so much pain I can't even think. My symptoms subside somewhat over November and December, giving me some reprieve to try to make up for the time I've lost.

In the meantime, BC Premier Gordon Campbell's Liberal government lays off tens of thousands of people from the civil service at the same time as Blair is trying to find some permanent work. He does piecemeal organizing work for social justice campaigns and finds very short-term, badly paying research work at the university. A friend of mine who works in a bookstore tells me that they're getting piles of resumés from ex-civil servants with master's degrees every day. Throughout the fall, Blair's out of work way more than he's in it.

If any one of these things hadn't happened, this story would have been drastically different. If the material that Mitzi asked for had actually existed, it wouldn't have mattered how little time I spent getting it. If Mitzi hadn't decided that she needed to take me under her wing and mother me, she wouldn't have taken it all so personally. If Tara hadn't been targeted, I wouldn't have been in the national media supporting her. If Mitzi's good friend hadn't been teaching my Thursday morning class, Mitzi wouldn't have known that I kept missing class because my morning bowel distress was often too intense to function with. If Blair had had reliable work, it wouldn't have been so urgent that I kept Mitzi's job. And, of course, if only I hadn't been so incredibly sick, I could have coped with it all.

I call my friend Dawn in Toronto from a pay phone in the university library. She's worried because I am describing dizziness and nausea—and even more worried that I am more focused on my guilt about "failing" Mitzi than I am about my own health. Dawn's impression is that I desperately want to be able to do this work and produce things for Mitzi, but somehow I can't. I am sick, and it is impossible to tell what is wrong and why I am still so ill.

Mitzi stops my pay without warning, even after I've already started making up my hours and successfully finding what very little material exists in the periodicals. The bottom line is that she thinks I have been lying about being sick and instead using her research money for nefarious activist purposes. She fires me. In the course of our dispute, she calls me irresponsible, accuses me of always having "excuses," and tells me that I'm "not very bright." It ends with her finally giving me enough work to finish the last six weeks of the term before Christmas. It's a small victory but still leaves me without the income I was expecting for the rest of the school year. One afternoon, she informs me that I can "never be a historian" because I tell her that using the microfilm machine for more than an hour at a time makes the world spin, resulting in vomit. At the time, I don't know why it does. The gravity of her voice when she informs me of this puzzles me — I have never declared any desire to *be a historian*. I just want to study history for a while.

When I go to speak to my department head, Mitzi has already spoken to her. The department head characterizes the disagreement as a "personality conflict" and reveals that Mitzi believes I have "other priorities." At this point, it's almost Christmas. I've already applied for holiday retail work, but Mitzi didn't fire me until after the stores had already finished hiring. The department head can't understand why I would want to work with someone when it's so clearly not a "good fit." I can't understand what part of *eating* and *paying rent* she doesn't get. It's as though at this particular institution the only graduate students they're accustomed to are those being bankrolled by wealthy parents. I don't tell her this; it's not something she'll likely get. The university policy is that if one research job doesn't "work out" while a student is still in the time frame of an employment contract, the department has to come up with other work to complete the contract. The department head insists that this doesn't apply to me because I'm studying part-time and should never have been hired in the first place. Over the winter holidays, I finish every last thing Mitzi asked me to do and submit it to her office.

When I look back at that year and try to see myself clearly, I just get fragmented pieces. I think in some core way, I was barely there. The twenty-two-year-old version of Julie is disintegrating, outwardly less and less present in the world as inwardly my bowel tissue literally eats me from the inside out. Gazing into the past and looking at my younger self, all I can see are ulcerations and terror.

I'm so consistently sick at this point that I decide our water is contaminated and boil everything for ten minutes before using it. We go down to Vancouver's Granville Island for New Year's Eve. Bobbie is doing an art installation. It's fun and lovely, and even watching the fireworks light up the low-level clouds over the bay is more funny and pretty than disappointing. Then, on the way back to the apartment, I have cramps so painful that I run the last stretch and somehow get to the toilet on time. For the first time—as I watch the toilet bowl filling with bloody diarrhea—I really believe there's a problem. Still, I'm not ready to deal with it. I go back downstairs and prepare drinks and snacks for our friends who are on their way over.

I spend the rest of the holidays and the first week of school unable to go anywhere. I get to the bus stop and have to rush home to reunite with the toilet. At this point, I feel officially broken. The deepest humiliation is discovering that my lack of income means I can't even get a line of credit from the bank without my parents' signatures. So four months after leaving home for the first time, insisting that I'm capable of supporting myself and can control my own finances and life, I'm calling home for a co-signer on a line of credit. The phone call is torturous. My mum is certain that I've done something to get myself fired, which is fair enough. It's certainly not beyond the scope of imagination that I could have. She wants the details of all my financial transactions before she'll consider signing anything. My dad finally gets on the phone and simply asks how much I was applying for on the line of credit and sends the cheque without question. I feel guilty but don't have much of a choice.

When I'm still not feeling any better, I heed Maia's and Blair's insistence that I see a doctor. I go back to the same walk-in clinic, and this time I see a woman. She's sympathetic but still just as dismissive.

"Oh, you're a graduate student, and you have two jobs, of course, you're stressed out. No wonder you have diarrhea. If there was something really wrong with you, you would have lost more weight. Blood? Here's a prescription for some hemorrhoid cream."

I figure, based on my own research, that I have ulcers that are best treated by natural means anyway. It is somewhat reassuring that she clearly doesn't think anything major is wrong with me. I start an ulcer diet, which does relieve the symptoms. At the same time, the new provincial government is making massive cuts to social programs, and in response, there are huge campaigns. Among all the things I attended, a memory sticks in my mind of joining the nurses' union and hospital employees' union picket across the street from the downtown hospital, outside of a hotel where the Ministry of Health is meeting. At the time, I have no clue that I'll meet these picketing health care professionals again in a very different context.

Organizing starts for the summer meeting of the G8 conference in Kananaskis, Alberta. The leaders of the eight richest countries in the world are getting together, and along with millions of others around the world, I'm motivated to get involved in protesting. I go out to Alberta for different meetings. I take an overnight bus ride to Canmore, Alberta, just after I put myself on the ulcer diet. Looking back, I can see it's kind of ridiculous. I'm extremely dizzy most of the time and experiencing muscle weakness. I'm secretly afraid of travelling alone, in case I pass out on the bus or something, but I'm pretty vague about this when I unsuccessfully try to talk people into coming with me. I guess that's the confusion intrinsic to denial—to deny that things aren't serious means some part of me must know they *are*, and yet, if I can't admit it to myself, I certainly can't ask other people for the support I need. The bus ride ends up going pretty smoothly, and I actually do have a great trip with awesome weather, and I meet lovely new people.

Blair finally finds a steady job. He'd been looking non-stop in all sorts of quarters since we arrived in Vancouver, so he's *thrilled* when he finds a job typing the phone book. He spends his days editing and inputting the telephone directory on a very temperamental and irrationally designed computer system. But the wages are reasonable, and higher than those of some people we know with computer-programming jobs, so things aren't so bad. I also start enjoying school. I'm taking a practicum course with Tara that involves interesting research, and our classroom seminars are engaging. The other students in the class are mixed between graduate and undergraduate, breaking down the competitive atmosphere I had unexpectedly encountered in my graduate seminars, where people seemed afraid to say what they actually thought in case it offended the wise professor. We openly discuss issues of activism and the academy—it's more like the far less pretentious environment I was accustomed to in my undergraduate degree. Tara is very encouraging and agrees to replace Mitzi as my supervisor.

Throughout this time, my chest infection repeatedly comes back. My system is so depleted I just can't get rid of common colds and flu. I also don't eat when I need to be somewhere important. We organize a campaign on campus against tuition fee hikes that hundreds of students get involved in. It culminates when we occupy the president's office the day and night before the scheduled board of governors' meeting, where the administration will decide how much to raise student fees. I don't eat for thirty-six hours for fear that it might bring on an attack. At this point, I'm so absorbed with what I need to do, and so convinced that nothing can be done medically about my poor digestion, that such extreme measures just seem like my only choice.

I go straight to Tara's evening class after we wrap up the occupation. Despite the lack of food and sleep, I'm feeling great. The new department chair is sitting in on our class. I've never met her before. For the purpose of this story, let's call her Snot-Face. I can't think of any other name for her; I have no generosity in my interpretation. She only ever revealed one dimension of herself to me, so that's the name she gets. I can see the look on Tara's face. She's telling me to stop talking about the occupation. But the lack of sleep and pure adrenalin rush of the last two days mean that I just can't. My mouth is out of my control; I'm excitedly bubbling over my own edges, leaking out excitement. Snot-Face just glares.

The month after this incident, we have a graduate student symposium. During the morning tea and cookies and schmooze fest, I walk past Mitzi and Snot-Face. It's hard to type this without part of me asking myself if I'm just making this up because it seems so unbelievable, but they literally snicker, whisper, and point at me as I walk by. During my panel, Mitzi slumps in her chair in the back of the room, wearing sunglasses. *Indoors.* She doesn't wear them for anyone else's presentation. If it occurred to me to put this in a novel, I'd probably decide that it's too over the top and that the characters' behaviour is too exaggerated and one-dimensional and I'd leave it out. And I'm incredulous as it happens. I'm pissed off too because their tactics actually do shake me. I hear my voice coming out of my mouth, unusually unsure, as I talk about the issues I'm now interested in pursuing for my thesis. Mitzi actually smirks from under her giant glasses. The fact that I've shifted my research so drastically seems to be proof that she was right. But I'm a twenty-two-year-old master's student. I thought the point was to explore and move in many directions and learn as much as possible from many perspectives and many people. I later hear from another student that Mitzi's had some major personal issues going on that year. I don't know if this is true; the other student barely knows her, she just reports friend-of-a-friend rumours and having personally repeatedly seen Mitzi in distress. I don't know where this fits into the puzzle of figuring out my blurry year in Vancouver, but maybe if Mitzi had been happier herself, she could've spared some compassion for me.

Two days later, I'm speaking at an activist conference in Victoria about G8 organizing. I'm so tired before my session that I fall asleep in the hallway. I'm embarrassed that someone might see me, so I keep waking myself up and plying myself with sugar and caffeine. I spend the ferry ride home locked in the toilet stall. As I gradually get worse, I get increasingly hard on myself. When I can't wake up in the morning, I believe I'm getting really lazy. When I can't concentrate or remember things, I decide that my intelligence is deteriorating. As my digestive symptoms worsen, I think it's my fault for not eating "right." Things that I normally find exciting or compelling become boring or too much trouble. When I imagine slitting my wrists, I tell myself that I'm pathetic and losing my mind. Things are spinning out of control. Part of me secretly thinks I'm probably dying of colon cancer, but I push this thought firmly away.

I return to Toronto to give a paper at an academic conference. I'm feeling very sick, with no energy at all, but I assume I'm coming down with the flu. My mum insists that I see my family doctor, and he hits the roof. He can't believe that the doctors I saw didn't send me to a gastroenterologist for tests. My flight back to Vancouver is the same week, so my doctor doesn't have time to get me the tests. Instead, he makes me promise that the day I get back I'll go to a different doctor and get a referral to a gastroenterologist. In the meantime, he says, "If you get a fever or chills, go straight to emergency."

Several days later, still in Toronto, I'm at another conference. I'm supposed to be giving a talk on the last day, but every time I sit down to try to organize my notes, all my thoughts are bleeding together and I can't focus. I'm constantly feeling very cold. I ask around. The room isn't cold. When I walk back to the place I'm staying, I can't stop shivering. My sister, Joanne, visits me that night. She's feeling my forehead and demanding that I go to the hospital. Part of the problem of being strong-willed and generally rational is that it is very easy to convince people that I'm thinking clearly when I'm most definitely not. My logic is that I'm too sick to move from the bed, too cold to go outside, and as such, certainly I can't leave to go to the hospital. And doesn't everyone know that I'm not really sick anyway? I'm convinced that I'm fooling everyone into believing something is wrong with me when I'm really just depressed and demoralized and wanting to stay in bed. Whether this is simply a delusion of the fever or an internalized interpretation of my mind and body based on eight months of disbelief and dismissal by academics and medical professionals is impossible to know.

6. Humble Resistance

My mum, my sister, and Blair gang up on me and take me to the hospital near my parents' house. I'm sitting in the emergency waiting room, huddled between Blair and my mum, still shivering. I have this endless desire to express; all I want to do is talk and talk and talk. They repeatedly ask me to stop with my desires for funeral arrangements and plans for Susie.

"What?" I say calmly. "No one expects to die suddenly. That's kind of the point."

I'm not consciously being morbid or melodramatic; I just want my wishes to be known. I'm so extreme. I go from *I'm not sick, I'm not sick, I'm just lazy and faking it* to *I'm dying* and back in a heartbeat. This back-and-forth lets me out of the truth: I have no control of this leaky mess. My body is doing what it's doing, and I have no idea what it means, what happens next, or how to stop it.

A nurse finally calls my name in a voice that makes me feel like a teenager who's been caught with a dirty room. Back in the high school years, I remember hiding under my bed covers, on the phone with my friend Kara, as my mum hovered outside, trying to suck me out to participate in some kind of cleaning activity. I dubbed this technique of my mother's the Nefarious Vacuum Voice. And now the nurse has it.

"Julie Devaney? Okay, this way..."

I earn my gurney. They wheel me into a flimsy, curtained space in the emergency ward, euphemistically described as Room 2. I spend six hours here with a dangerously high fever, near hallucination. I make up silly songs with Blair about wanting someone to come to Room 2 to talk about my poo. I decide that I'm moving back to Toronto after the summer. I feel defeated; Vancouver has done this to me.

When the nurses are finally able to get the doctor to see me, he is furious.

"How was she left lying here for six hours in this state? How did she get into this state?" He turns to me. "You've had bloody diarrhea for *how* long and you didn't think to see a doctor?"

"About six months, and I saw two different ones—three times. They said the blood was hemorrhoids and the diarrhea was just stress."

"And you believed them?"

He's incredulous and yelling at me. During his outraged interrogation, four nurses and another doctor desperately try to find a vein hydrated enough to start an intravenous line. A note to future doctors: if you're going to fire off questions at patients with critically high fevers, wait until they answer the first question before making accusations in the second. Also, please don't encourage us to question the diagnosis or lack thereof of your colleagues—it will only get us into trouble in future dealings with your establishment.

My blood work reveals anemia and dangerously low levels of sodium and potassium: all contributors to fatigue, dizziness, nausea, lack of concentration, memory loss, and depression. Things are starting to make a little more sense.

I am admitted to Room 604, which is, somewhat appropriately, the Vancouver area code. The next morning, the gastroenterologist, Dr. Lane, manages to get a room and technicians to perform a scope, even though it's Sunday. It's the day I am scheduled to give my conference talk. Instead, I watch on the TV screen as Dr. Lane pushes the camera through my bloody, mangled colon, with massive, pus-filled holes oozing on the sides. She decides that instead of giving me any anaesthetic she'll use paediatric tools, and then it won't hurt. It won't hurt her, but for me, it's excruciating. The psychological trauma of seeing the insides of my body so diseased combines with the physical agony. I can see the faces of every person who was vicious and nasty to me in Vancouver reflected out of each bubbling pool of pus.

An anaesthetist has come and really wants to give me sedation, but my doctor insists that it isn't necessary. Her rationale is that if I'm medicated, it will be *more* of an ordeal for me because it'll take longer for me to recover and longer before I can go back to my room and see my mum and Blair. The anaesthetist holds my hand and says, "Oh, honey," every time I moan and gasp in pain. My doctor doesn't hide her professional excitement witnessing the oozing evidence supporting her diagnosis.

"Yes, yes, that's definitely ulcerative colitis. See that, Julie — the inflammation, the ulcerations, the mucus, the bleeding. See how the disease is consistent, no patches. We'll just take a little snip here for the biopsy. Just one more. Well, you're doing great, Julie, just great. You're doing great."

I gasp again in response. And then it's over, and a porter pushes me back to my room.

When I get back to my room and tell my mum and Blair Dr. Lane's diagnosis, much to my surprise, my mum says, "That's what I have."

"Ulcerative colitis? Really? I thought you had IBS, irritable bowel syndrome."

"No," she corrects me. "IBD, inflammatory bowel disease. I was diagnosed about five years ago. I thought you knew."

"But you never seemed that sick..."

"I wasn't," she agrees. "They just put me on some mild medication, and it settled down."

This revelation becomes my new source of hope. If my mother's disease was managed so easily, surely mine could be too.

The following morning a male nurse comes in with a "hat" to take a stool sample. I go into the washroom, lift the seat, place the hat down, lower the seat, and poo into the hat. The hat fills with blood, and I leave it there to go and tell the nurse that the sample is ready.

He immediately comes back out of the washroom, not bothering to hide his frustration.

"You weren't supposed to *pee* in the hat."

"I didn't," I tell him.

It turns out that pushing a camera through my diseased colon massively increased my bleeding. It seems somewhat predictable to me. So I have daily injections of vitamin K added to my hospital regimen to stop the bleeding.

My first hospital stay is more than entertaining. I have three roommates: Mrs. Taylor, Peggy, and Lena. Peggy is an older lady in the bed directly across from me. She's very popular, and the phone is usually for her, though the rest of the time it's always for me. Every time it rings, she yells, "Julie, your turn!" to get me to answer it.

Mrs. Taylor is in the bed to her right, so diagonally across from me. She's having some kind of respiratory problem. Every night, several times a night, she removes her respirator and calls out in a pained and wheezing voice, "Jesus! Sweet Jesus, take me nowww! Jeee-sss-uuusss!!"

I start the nightly ritual in which my roommates dutifully take their turn, of buzzing the nurses' station and saying, mimicking the hospital pages, "Mrs. Taylor for Jesus, Bed 2, Mrs. Taylor, looking for Jesus to take her, Bed 2." Or when we're really tired, with a yawn, "Mrs. Taylor wants Jesus to take her...again..."

I am by far the youngest of any patients I see. The guy delivering the food trays points this out.

"You're too young to be here!" he says while sympathizing about the general lack of food in the clear fluids diet the doctors have me on.

I tell him, "I have colitis; any food at all is exciting compared to barely eating at all, which is what I was doing before I got here."

"Oh," he says, understanding. "You're a GI patient."

GI Julie. The title appeals to me.

During this hospital stay I decide that nurses are superhuman ether-beings delivered from another planet to save us all. At the same time, I always feel indebted to them for everything they do. I am hyper-conscious that they are working a very difficult job, and want to make myself as little trouble as possible. Strategically, this also seems wise because of how completely helpless I feel as a patient. Better to keep the nurses sweet. Practically, it seems a bit counterintuitive, a kind of compulsion to take care of my caregivers.

On my second-to-last day, my favourite nurse, Margarita, takes me to the shower. As we walk down the wide open hallway, I realize my gown is flapping open at back. I self-consciously clutch at it to cover my bare bum. She looks behind me.

"If I had an ass like that," she says, "I'd show it off."

I laugh, pleased. I don't really believe her at the time, but looking back with a more gentle and generous gaze, I think she might have meant it.

When I get back from the shower, I have a splitting headache. Since being admitted three days earlier, I haven't really gotten any sleep. The warmth of the shower and the peace of the afternoon lull me to sleep.

I am abruptly awakened by Preacher Nurse. She roughly cuffs my arm to read my blood pressure. She doesn't speak to me except to say, "Praise God," and continue muttering her liturgy. The pain of my migraine and the complete vulnerability I feel is intense. And now I wake up from my first real sleep by someone hurting my arm while talking to God. It brings on my first tears. I hold my breath until she leaves, and then I sob and sob.

Margarita sticks her head in. "What's wrong, honey? What's the matter?"

"My head hurts," I cry.

She gets me cool cloths and comforts me, rubbing my arm until I go back to sleep. Suddenly, I've reverted from being an adult to being everyone's "honey." It's strange how sometimes it's the smallest things that wouldn't ordinarily faze me that make me crack, and the attempts at coddling that would generally make me cringe are exactly what I need.

Then I am itching to prove I'm well enough to leave.

"Great, great. I'm great; everything's great," I say whenever Dr. Lane comes in. She gives me a "bowel chart" to fill in. I keep it at the side of my bed, and after every movement, I amuse myself by using colourful words and graphic detail. At various points, the words "black forest cake," "Guinness," and "CSI" are all in play. The movements are becoming fewer and there's less blood and mucus in them.

Apparently I've also contracted a bad urinary tract infection since I arrived in the ER. It's supposed to be very painful, so all the doctors and nurses are surprised that I haven't even noticed it. I think there's only a certain amount of pain and discomfort that my body can register, and then it just doesn't bother telling me about the rest.

When Peggy goes home, Lena asks to switch so she's next to the window, across from me. Less than half a day passes before Pauline is brought in, wearing restraints and with two police officers keeping watch at the door. It's hard to know exactly what is going on except that the woman separated from me by a curtain clearly doesn't want to be there. She wants a cigarette, she does not want a hospital gown, and she does not want to be touched. Because of the security risk she supposedly represents, she's not even allowed up to use the washroom. Our entire room stinks of bedpan waste, and Lena and I secretly pass perfume back and forth to mask the smell.

Pauline insists that she doesn't know what happened and why she's there. As the night progresses, we listen to the conversations she has with the nurses. She woke up in emergency, restrained on a stretcher. Her last memory is sitting on her couch with a headache and taking some Tylenol. She's certain she didn't overdose. Apparently, when her daughter came home, Pauline was unconscious, and the paramedics assumed it was a suicide attempt. No one believes her. The next morning, a psychiatrist walks in with a spring in his step and a forced grin on his face.

He surveys the room, settles on me, and walks confidently to my bed. "Pauline?" he asks.

"No!" I reply.

He mutters an apology, looks at the bed numbers, and sits down next to Pauline.

Finally, the truth comes out. "Your blood report came back, Pauline. It turns out you really did just take a Tylenol."

I don't know why they have sent a mental health professional to tell her this. As if there's something odd about reacting with the venom she did when waking up bolted to a stretcher in an emergency ward where no one believes a word you say. I wonder how the doctor would be acting if he spent the night tied to a bed using a bedpan with police at the door.

"Do you have a history of seizures, Pauline?" he asks.

"I told them that I do," she replies, now sounding weak and battle-weary. "Yes, I've had seizures in the past."

"Okay, then," he says. "We'll get you a neurologist."

Why no one got her a neurologist as soon as she came in, unconscious on a stretcher with a history of seizures, is a matter I can only speculate on. My guess is that when the paramedics brought in a working-class black woman who'd been passed out on her couch with no immediate explanation, the emerg doctor just assumed she'd been abusing substances. Why waste precious resources and the time of prestigious specialists when she probably just did it to herself? Not the most scientific approach to the situation. I'm furious for her but definitely not feeling well enough to get involved. It also occurs to me how much easier it is for me to become infuriated on someone else's behalf than on my own.

I get that the emerg doctors did not have any information when she arrived in the ambulance—but it seems to me that when an extreme protocol involving restraints and police guards gets put into place in a clinical context, there should be an opportunity for a patient to clarify the situation. It seems that nothing Pauline said or did to contradict their assumptions was given any weight. Once the medical professionals had put the process in motion, only blood tests and psychiatrists were given the authority to tell her story—her words, however true, were considered unreliable.

Dr. Lane comes in to discharge me a few hours later. She prescribes some special bowel anti-inflammatory and iron for the anemia. I've learned in the books that there are two different inflammatory bowel diseases: ulcerative colitis (UC) and Crohn's disease. The prognosis is much better for UC because it only affects the colon, whereas Crohn's disease can manifest anywhere in the entire digestive tract, from mouth to anus.

The oral medications are working, and they're still very mild compared with the other steroid and immune medications I read about in the book. I feel mostly optimistic because at least I understand what's going on, yet I am still shaken by the ordeal of being hospitalized.

Within the week, I am back at my parents' house and feeling better than I have in a really long time. Diagnosis with a chronic illness is supposed to be traumatic. For me, it's a giant relief. I finally know what's wrong; it has a name, and apparently it's not my fault.

Now I'm in the "everybody's an expert" phase of illness. Where people I don't even like feel empowered to approach me with unsolicited advice.

"I heard you have ulcers. My uncle had ulcers. He didn't have to go to the hospital though. I know it's painful, but it's okay; you'll get over it."

"I used to have digestive problems. Then I stopped eating dairy and red meat. You should try that."

"You take care of yourself. Make sure you eat right and exercise."

I treat this phase with extreme impatience.

"Are you sure you have to take all that medication? Have you tried any natural methods?"

"Young people these days, popping pills for everything...I haven't even taken an aspirin for a headache in ten years."

For one thing, it's the kind of judgmental moralism I spent my youth resisting in Catholic school. For another thing, it's patronizing and offensive. *No, I've never thought of "eating right." Exercise? I prefer video games and daytime television. The "toilet sprint" is the only track and field event I've been capable of lately.*

Someone I don't know very well reveals to me that her husband has ulcerative colitis. I immediately open up to her, confiding that I'm feeling anxious and stressed about having a relapse. She immediately reprimands me.

"Don't do that. That's what makes you sick—stress. Just don't let yourself think that way. I'm positive that that's what this disease is all about: negative thinking."

When I'm in the mood, I address the medical confusion directly, correcting people. When I'm feeling ambushed, at parties, for example, I get a bit passive-aggressive.

"You know, since I became ill, people have been giving me all kinds of advice. Do you know what I say to them?"

"No, what?" asks the innocent and well-meaning friend.

"You're not my fucking doctor."

He looks shocked and hurt, but I really don't care. Most people get the point, but there are always a few who persist.

My family doesn't even want me to finish the summer in Vancouver. My dad repeatedly reminds me that there are lots of indispensable people in the graveyard, which looks harsher in print than it sounds out loud. He doesn't actually think I'm going to die; he just thinks that Vancouver would survive without me. But I feel compelled to finish what I begin. So I'm going back to Vancouver for three months and then moving to Toronto. The story I tell at the time is that Dr. Lane, my gastroenterologist, is completely insistent that I need to move back for treatment.

But this isn't strictly true. I really want to be home in Toronto. I'm terrified of staying in Vancouver. But I'm even more afraid that people will be mad at me or judge me for giving up. So I've already made the decision before I ask Dr. Lane the very leading question.

"I really shouldn't stay in Vancouver, should I? Do you think I should move back?"

To which she emphatically answers, "Yes! Get out of Vancouver!"

And I exhale a great sigh of relief.

7. Pinko in Paris

I'm flashing forward to prettier times. It's summer 2006. The first time in five years I've spent six consecutive months having more healthy days than sick ones. I've finally completed all the coursework for my master's degree, successfully held down a job organizing a conference, and just performed the earliest version of my show for the first time. The fantasy I nurtured through hospitalizations and health policy lectures of getting into my gown and performing scenes from my stretcher at the front of classrooms has finally become a reality. I'm writing my thesis, which is now based on my illness writings and performances. My supervisor for my new master's program in Toronto, Margrit, keeps giving me great things to read. For the first time since I was a small child, I'm a student with no commitments other than school—and now a comfortable, mostly healthy body as well.

I start a blog and call it *The Pinko Julie Show*, with the tagline "political in pink." My idea is that I'll tell my stories in real time, as if narrating scenes from my life as they're happening. I want it to be less a space of reflection and more of one where pieces of my life are being played out as if they're on a stage or a screen. Beginning completely anonymously, I reveal my identity piece by piece until I'm stripped naked—exposed to the world. Like every creative project I've ever done, the way it ultimately turns out is completely unpredictable at the outset. For one thing, in the surge of energy and excitement that spurred me to begin, I secretly expect instant fame and superstardom.

I travel from Toronto, to Washington, DC, to the UK for performances. The conferences I applied to in the fall—when I ran out of patience with writing and talking about chronic illness from a detached academic perspective—have unexpectedly all welcomed me to come and perform. At first I'm horrified; I didn't anticipate that they would all say yes. I'm also scared to travel on my own. I used to fly all the time and loved airplanes, but now it feels all new again. Then, when I arrive, I feel the strength in my legs; I feel the relief of comfort and ease in my abdomen, the tingle of excitement in my chest. I am alive, I am well, and I am ready for new adventures. The *joy* of being in my body and travelling in the sun after spending so long isolated in the dark is incredible. I perform to a classroom of people at a conference in England, and then move on to visit old friends and meet new ones. I feel like I'm emerging from the longest winter of my life, fresh and renewed, blooming into spring. Exposing myself to the world, and the world to me.

I go to Paris for a few days to visit my friend Caro. She's writing her dissertation, so the plan is for me to entertain myself in places other than her apartment during the day and for us to meet up in the evening. I'm not always great with directions, but in Paris, I feel like I've known these streets forever. I wander comfortably, loosely around the streets and on and off the metro. I find myself at major tourist attractions and hidden laneway cafés.

I blog:

> I quickly decide that in my short visit, I do not want to go to
> any galleries, museums, or tourist attractions. The weather
> is beautiful, my host is willing to take me out in the evenings
> with her friends, so during the day I just want to walk around

and pretend to be French. Paris is the most luscious and beautiful reward after a very long trek.

I wander through the streets, looking at the areas I've read about, soaking in the outdoor art, architecture, fashion. I try on very, very expensive clothes. I count how many people ask me for directions in French. I stop for lunch in a picturesque cafe. It is right on the corner of a fantastic intersection with a great view...

The thing I'm really loving about Paris is the live art. Watching the way people interact with their environment and seeing the scenes change. I imagine the ways I can recreate the high fashions with cheaper clothes and realize that I won't really be motivated to do so when I leave. But it's fun nonetheless. I don't want to do any overtly tourist things until the very last morning before I leave. I decide then that I can leave my pretensions behind for an hour-long boat tour along the Seine. It's well worth it. But my favourite moment is still the simplest. Standing in Marais with my friend, waiting for her friends to show up, eating a falafel, and feeling like I'm having an authentic Parisian moment.

Late into the night, we sit in Caro's apartment with the lights off, watching scenes unfold in the apartments across the street. We drink wine and watch and chat and imagine scenarios as if they're in a soap opera. I think about the fact that if we weren't sitting there, no one would see these moments. Would we be any less connected in this exquisite web if they had gone unobserved? On this trip, I experience a new bodily freedom that I haven't had in the past five years. I can travel alone, feel healthy, not be scared. My body is a site of pleasure, and it's all mine. Not vulnerable to health care professionals, medical side effects, and hospital rules.

I go back to the UK and stay with Bobbie in Manchester. We end up participating in an art installation. She's living in an artists' co-op at the time that frequently hosts people who are in town to put on various shows and exhibits. At breakfast, we get talking to a group of Scottish artists who are doing a live-art piece in a centuries-old indoor swimming pool nearby. The water is ice cold. They've put an inflatable, oversized 1950s Space Age-looking device in the middle of the pool and invited the general public to come swimming and play on the floaty platform.

They ask us if we'd be willing to wear silver bathing suits they've brought and be filmed. So we go along. I dive into the freezing water in my silver suit and swim to the middle. In the coming weeks, they have an exhibit in a Manchester gallery. I've left by then but hear from Bobbie that the clip of me diving is on permanent loop at the entrance to the show. And as usual, I find myself at a political demonstration. As it wraps up, I blog:

> As I sit down against a tree, people start piling placards on either side of me. I notice someone with a camera taking my picture. I'm not sure if he wants the natural look of an exhausted protester looking off at the crowd until he yells, "Smile for the camera." Amused with myself for being so concerned about my cool, nonchalant pose, I grin at him, laughing. "Nice one!" he shouts as he captures the shot. He smiles, waves, and walks off. I wonder what's going to happen to the picture and think about all the ways we float in and out of each other's lives. Constantly connecting and disconnecting. I look up at the crowd again: families, youth, older people, activists, people who have never been on demonstrations before in their lives. I feel connected.

8. Dr. Cartoon

Back in my summer of bodily breakdown in Vancouver, I'm still falling apart—feeling disconnected, alienated. I decide to do a reading course in the summer while organizing for the G8 protests in Alberta. My troubles seem small compared to an AIDS pandemic in Africa and a looming war in Iraq. The eight most powerful men in the world are going to be meeting one province away, and we're organizing buses to go and protest.

My schedule feels a lot more manageable, and I start believing that everything will be fine. Tara is now my master's supervisor, and she's being incredibly supportive. Within a week, I get my first period since my diagnosis. The symptoms come back with a rage, and the pain is worse than it has ever been. I am terrified that I am actually having potentially fatal complications in the middle of the night when my entire body is in spasm from the pain. Blair gets me into a cab and we head to Vancouver General. The triage nurse asks me, as I am doubled over in tears with pain, to rate my pain on a scale of one to ten. My pain is definitely a ten, but I want to imagine that there could be worse pain, somewhere, somehow. So I say, "nine point five." I'm not sure why it is that in the throes of terrifying pain I feel the need to use decimals. The rationale isn't conscious at the time, but in retrospect, I can't help wondering if it's some deep-rooted desire to expose the absurdity of trying to put a numerical digit on my pain. They immediately put me on a stretcher and give me Demerol and Gravol intravenously. Finally, peace washes over my body.

It's short-lived. A young resident physician comes in and, within seconds, pronounces, "You've been misdiagnosed. You have a serious case of Crohn's disease. We're going to need to put you on intravenous steroids. You might be here for weeks."

The specialist joins them. With oversized glasses and clothes, he looks more like a cartoon character than a person. He dismissively tells me that my brilliant doctor in Toronto—whom I'm deeply in love with—was wrong.

"The medication she gave you was like trying to treat a house fire with a drip of water instead of a hose."

I survey the two men peering down at me with their crossed arms. The big men are here to take out the steroidal hose. Dr. Cartoon looks excited at the prospect of doing a scope.

A nurse comes into my enclave with the pre-scope enema. Three walls, one curtain. I can't reach the curtain.

"Do you want me to do it?" she asks reluctantly. "Or can you just do it yourself?"

I've never even seen an enema bottle before, much less performed an enema on myself.

"Can you do it?" I ask weakly, lying prone on the stretcher.

She complies, and then when I protest that I can't hold it in, she says with a sigh, "Well, just let it out then. Unless you think you can make it to the bathroom."

The potential indignity of soaking my bed outweighs my doubts about the seemingly impossible feat of traversing the ER dragging an IV pole while keeping my flapping gown closed at the back. The nurse casually watches as I embark on this humiliating venture of resistance. I manage to hold the liquid in by sheer force of will until I reach the toilet that's at the complete opposite end of the ward.

When I get back, I insist to everyone who will listen that I need pain medication and sedation. Short of breaking into a rendition of "I Wanna Be Sedated" by the Ramones (which I later do privately for Blair), I can't possibly be more explicit.

When I tell Dr. Cartoon that I need to be well medicated because my last scope was horrible, he laughs loudly, throwing his head back and repeating, "Horrible?"

"Yes!" I say. "Horrible!"

I feel myself being wheeled into the scope room, where they give me a small dose of Valium. It seems they're of the just-shut-the-woman-up school, seeing as Valium has no effect whatsoever on my pain; it just purports to be vaguely calming. As they push the camera back through my inflamed and bleeding rectum and sigmoid colon (now for the second time in several weeks), I tell them, "Owww, this is really, really hurting. This is extremely painful."

Their conversation with one another doesn't miss a beat. I scream, but it doesn't break their rhythm.

"Oh, it doesn't look that bad; the medication seems to be working. Her diagnosis is correct. Send her home."

The doctors vacillate between extremes — it's either "You'll be in here for weeks" or it's complete dismissal — without addressing the intense pain I arrived with and without providing any opportunity for discussion.

And so they send me home with a prescription for steroid enemas and an appointment with Dr. Cartoon in a month. I have absolutely no trust in the motives and skills of this doctor. I feel like I have been assaulted by a gang of men in white coats. They can prove quite easily that I consented. The paperwork bears my signature. But who feels free to refuse medical treatment while being pushed through an emergency room? What's consensual about agreeing to a procedure that is posed as your only treatment option while vast amounts of pain are consuming you?

Dr. Cartoon doesn't bother to see me again before I'm discharged but passes the message along that I no longer need to take iron supplements because my hemoglobin is high enough and I am no longer anemic. To me, this does not physically seem to be true. I still feel weak and look very pale. But I accept that if my hemoglobin is within the lab's range of normal, it must be fine. I conclude that if my oral anti-inflammatories appear to be working and the scope revealed that my disease was contained in my rectum and very end of my sigmoid colon, the best first option is the same medication in suppository form. I want to at least explore this possibility before taking these enemas that I haven't been shown how to use and that, because of their steroid content, are only supposed to be used under close supervision of a medical professional. I'm also terrified of the directions that come in the box. They describe risks of tearing and all manner of other side effects. The only medical professional I really trust at his point is Dr. Lane in Toronto.

I go back to the walk-in clinic that had diagnosed me with "stress." I want to throw my real diagnosis in the doctor's face and see if I can get my medication in suppositories—and also get a referral to a non-abusive gastroenterologist who at least attempts to demonstrate some basic humanity. When I tell the doctor who'd said I was "just stressed out" about my last couple of months, she feels terrible. She prescribes me the medication I request but is concerned that she can't find me another specialist because the shortest wait time for an appointment is three months, and I'll already be back in Toronto by then. I ask to see my blood results from the test she did in January. My hemoglobin was twenty points higher than it was in the hospital test earlier in the week. She tells me that it shouldn't fluctuate more than five points, so what was normal for the hospital lab was not normal for me. I start taking the iron again.

Two days later, I'm on a panel about the G8 that packs out the Vancouver public library. It's really fun, and my meds seem to be working again. I missed the prep meeting the day I had been hospitalized, and when I say I wasn't there because I was ill, one of the organizers flippantly responds, "Yeah, nobody feels well."

I don't think he's trying to be mean, just agreeing that everyone's coming down with things. But I feel like he's just slapped me. The dilemma that has torn me in two since the onset of this illness is how tempting it is to throw the severity of what I've gone through out at people and make them choke in contrast with the horrific sensation associated with how I imagine people seeing me as a "sick" person—just that shade less than human, other, different, not quite credible or whole.

So I stay quiet.

My health is still really up and down. Some days, I feel fine and can participate in the world, and other days I'm incapacitated again. We go to the G8 protests in Calgary, and I feel a bit more fragile than usual but strengthened and cheered up by the bright and lively demonstrations. When we get home, I get sicker and sicker. I just want to hold out until the move back to Toronto. Just want to finish one more reading course, organize one more meeting. As Blair watches me deteriorate, he starts screening my calls. I hear him in the other room interrogating my friends, "Are you calling to ask how she's feeling? Because she's in bed; she's not well. So, no politics, nothing that's going to stress her out."

Before my illness, it was completely out of character for Blair to be so direct. He keeps his tone light as if he's teasing, but he clearly means it. And he's right: many of the calls were about things that would've definitely stressed me out if he hadn't set such strict parameters. During this flare-up, my joints start to hurt and my toilet frequency increases to twelve times a day, with cramping excruciating enough to make me throw up. It's hard to describe how frightening it feels to have my body produce so much pain that I lose control. In the moment, it's impossible to believe it will ever end. Sometimes I clutch the bathroom walls or turn the taps on hot and cold and scorch or freeze my hands, just wincing and moaning, trying to do anything to distract myself from the pain. I always put the fan on, as well as the taps, just to make sure no one hears me cry out. It's so difficult for me to be natural and open when communicating pain and distress to other people. My automatic reaction is always to cover it up with a veneer of casual ease and calm. When I do express it, I feel like an actor in a play. It's not quite this explicit in my conscious mind at the time, but it's almost as if some part me is asking, *If someone else was having this experience how might they act? What might they say? How would they convey their feelings to their friends and loved ones?* And so when I do say these things and act these ways, I feel like a fraud, and the part of me that always secretly believes that I'm "faking" is vindicated. To get to the point where it's possible for anyone to convince me to go to the hospital is the point where I am really at rock bottom.

In this middle-of-the-night trip, we take a cab downtown to avoid Dr. Cartoon at the hospital close to home.

9. Leaky Hospitals

The emergency ward in Vancouver's downtown hospital is literally leaking bodies. Before the *snap!* of the glove on the Vancouver emergency doctor's hand, this is how things look:

I'm leaning against the wall of the ER, in front of the triage desk, trying to give the person talking to the nurse some privacy. A woman comes in on a stretcher, crying, her partner hovering anxiously at her side. In my memory, there's blood on the white sheets between her legs, but I can't know if that's true. I might have just heard that she'd had a miscarriage and added that detail in my imagination. Two kids, obviously high on something, are telling the nurse that their legs hurt, or their chests, or they're not sure. They just walked and walked, and one became sure that one of his limbs was falling off. The other is now convinced that this limb detachment disease is contagious and that he has just caught it.

As I look around, I notice security approaching the teenagers. It seems to me that there are at least triple the number of security guards as there are medical staff. There's only one nurse running the triage station. I wonder how many security issues could be prevented if people could access treatment as soon as they walked in, agitated, sick, and scared.

A man in a business suit rushes in, running straight up to triage desk, pretending he doesn't see me waiting. Blair goes and stands next to him. As soon as the triage nurse becomes free, he starts talking frantically. I don't hear what he's saying, but Blair pushes me forward with his arm around me and says to the man, "She was here first."

The nurse is very sympathetic and immediately gets me a stretcher next to the window, with a curtain separating me from the rest of the ward. Blair tells me later that the man who shoved past us was complaining about a toothache. Two nurses, Wendell and Wendy, come to my stretcher and start talking to me. They joke about their matching names and how I must think I'm at the circus, making me laugh while they animatedly look for somewhere on my arms to start an IV. They call another nurse over, and he starts smacking the inside of my forearm, looking to see if a vein rises to the occasion.

"Stop it!" yells Wendell, horrified. "You're hurting her!"

"It's okay," I reply seriously. "It's a welcome distraction from the pain in my abdomen."

I am being completely truthful and only mildly ironic, but they're unsure whether to laugh or not. They find a vein and start my IV. Shortly after this chaotic entrance, I meet the exhausted emerg doctor and ultimately find myself stored in a closet, my body leaking out of the bounds of space intended for patients.

And as it turns out, my experience is hardly unique. More recently, I travelled back to British Columbia to perform and give a workshop for a Health Research Network. Right after the evening performance, Blair and I join some of the event organizers for dinner at a Mexican restaurant.

We're drinking sangria and waiting for food when Eliane, the director of the organization, turns to me and says, "You know, my friend was in your closet."

I'm amazed. "Really? When?"

"A few years ago. When were you in there?"

"In 2002, so probably still a few years before your friend. Why was she there?"

"Well, the whole thing was just a really terrible story. But she ended up in that particular closet because she was pregnant at the time, and the nurses felt really sorry for her. They wanted to protect her from the chaos of the ward. So, after all the trauma of her experiences, it was a safe space for her."

I'm amazed because I always use my closet story to illustrate the severity of the cutbacks and the indignity of my stretcher experiences. And it certainly is all these things. But there's something powerful, six years later, to hear that those nurses were looking out for me.

I don't remember how or when I get out of that closet and into a bed in a room. The scenes blur into grey swirling shadows that I can't quite grasp. But there are still crisp moments that light up in Technicolor. Nightmares I still haven't managed to wake up from. The massive amount of intense detail I've stored about particular moments is taking up all the memory in my neurological hard drive, like vivid short films that are individually meaningless but evocative in context—memories laid out like art installations.

Video art clips:

Waking up to the naked old woman trying to claw up the side of my bed as she pees on the floor, and the nurse, a tiny young woman, trying in vain to pull her back to her bed. This clip repeats on permanent loop.

Coming back from the washroom in the hall in the middle of the night and the nurse coming in to do my vitals. She's the nice one who microwaves bags of saline solution for me to put on my abdomen, getting around the rule against hot water bottles and heating pads.

She looks at me with shock and says, "Did you just walk out to the washroom?"

"Yes," I reply.

"And you felt okay?"

"Why?" I ask. "What's wrong?"

She rushes into the hall without answering.

Two different nurses come back. They each take an arm and look at their watches, counting out loud. They both get thirty-eight.

"What does that mean?" I demand.

"Does your chest hurt?"

"Yes, I've been having chest pain for a while. I'm finding it a bit difficult to breathe..."

"Open your mouth. We're just going to spray something onto your tongue. It's called nitroglycerine."

My mind is immediately taken to the scene in the British soap *Coronation Street* where Jack Duckworth is rushed into the ER with chest pain and they spray the inside of his mouth because he's having a *heart attack*. An article I read recently flashes into a freeze-frame on the inside of my forehead, consuming my imagination: *Young women are so statistically unlikely to go into cardiac arrest that it frequently goes undiagnosed.*

The resident on call rushes in at that point, hair messy, with a deliberately casual sort of just-woke-up air about him. He checks my heartbeat with his stethoscope.

"What's wrong with me?" I ask emphatically.

He forces a smile. "Oh, probably nothing."

No one explains. Everyone speaks with such forced serenity and false cheer that I think, *This must be what happens just before you die.*

Lying there in my hospital bed in the dark, I call upon my closet bunkmate to join me once again.

"Tommy!"

Nothing.

I try again. "Tommy, where are you?"

Still nothing. I close my eyes tightly and try to will him into existence. I think, *Maybe if I flex every muscle in my body, I will develop magical powers.* I use all my physical might to summon him.

No Tommy.

I fight back tears as I start drifting off to sleep, when suddenly, *Thud!* A form abruptly lands immediately to my left, narrowly missing my hip. I jar awake.

"Tommy?" I ask.

"Yes, I'm here. It's not the easiest thing to materialize, you know."

Just as he was when he flew into my closet, he's neatly dressed in a perfectly pressed suit.

"That's weird," I say. "How do you transcend space and time and look so pristine?"

"Magic," he replies.

10. Welcome Back, Tommy

As usual, I have dozens of questions for him. But first, I want to bring him up to speed.

"Tommy, I think my heart might stop beating. I hate it here. I'm probably going to die."

"Oh, Julie, you really need to get some sleep."

"This is true. But before I do, please, please, please tell me how we're going to sort this whole mess out."

He laughs sympathetically. "It always seems so impossible to change things. When you're in the middle of something it seems like it's the only way and that ordinary people can never impact these big systems. But I'm here to tell you—you already are changing the world."

I smile. "Thanks, but I have trouble believing that right here, right now. And every time we try to make any argument about why we need to save and protect public health care, they make all kinds of big claims about it costing too much."

Tommy interjects loudly, "I've heard the argument about health care costing *too much*, and it honestly confounds me. At what point in human history did someone decide that our ethical stances and values should be dictated by economic systems that *we* created?" At this point, he stands on my bed, hands emphatically gesturing in front of him. "There's nothing *natural* or *permanent* about the market; it's such a recent invention in our history. How about we first prioritize what we care about as a society and *then* create economic systems to support it?" His voice is booming at this point, but somehow my hospital roommates continue to sleep soundly. I look nervously at the doorway to see if any nurses are hovering. But Tommy is unfazed.

He continues. "Money should neither be a barrier to anyone accessing care, *nor* a way to buy superior quality of care. If we truly believe that all people are equal, then our health care system is the bottom line in making this a reality."

I see a soft light emanating from his fingertips, swirling around the room and surrounding us all in sparkling yellows and greens.

"Good night, Tommy," I say.

"Good night, Julie, and dream no little dreams…"

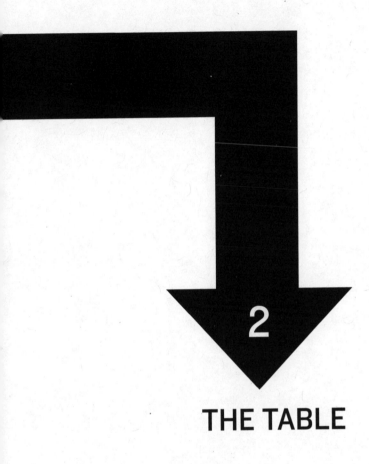

2

THE TABLE

I. An Education in Julie

"I heard you had a bad night" is the first thing the nurse says to me the next morning. Apparently "in good spirits" is no longer the defining comment on my chart.

A young resident comes in and sits in the chair beside me. She places her hand softly on my knee. I think she means it. I am so invested in mothering and encouraging the med students that I can forget what I need. I always tell her what a good job she's doing. She has small, delicate hands. An engagement ring and a wedding band. Well made-up, dyed blond hair. She could be on *90210*. She's the first person who seems at all concerned with the perennial burning in my urethra, despite a series of negative tests for urinary tract infections.

She and her friend take me downstairs for a pelvic exam. It's the last day, and I've been chatting with her so casually every time she comes to see me that when she asks if I want a wheelchair, I say no. It's almost funny because we just finished talking about the fact that my heart rate went down to thirty-eight beats per minute the night before, but because my voice is still commanding and my demeanour convincing, she agrees. It's a good few paces down the hall before the two of them realize that a wheelchair is most certainly necessary. And so they push me down into the examining room.

It's almost surreal: two women who easily could be my friends inserting a metal speculum into my vagina, asking if I'm sexually active. A discussion we should be having with laughter and wine, now pathologized into concerns about sexually transmitted diseases. A male med student walks in to complain that he needs the room. The two women groan, complaining that they had this room booked. Strange things happen when memories bleed together. Male interns and residents, for example, in different cities and different hospitals, all end up looking the same. They are all just screaming with insecurity, social awkwardness, and messy hair. I want to coddle them, fix their hair, then smack them, hard.

When the cardiologist comes in, he tells his residents what happened to me in words that I find indecipherable. All of my self-taught Latin about bowel disease and its extra-intestinal side effects are of no use in penetrating his lecture. When he leaves, a resident stays to update my chart.

"I don't understand," I tell him. "Can you explain what happened?"

He shows me the printout from the cardiogram. I can't even attempt to type the dialogue here because what he says still makes very little sense to me. Something about the heart having quarters, or ventricles or something, and for some reason one of mine slowed down. Now it's fine and it probably won't do it again. That's honestly the best I can do.

My mum phones frequently. While I was in the closet, she had such a hard time getting through. In one series of missteps, the phone got passed between so many nurses looking for me that my mum thought she heard them say I was in a coma. So when I give her the vague and inconsistent story about my heart rate, she panics. My dad gets on the phone and calmly explains that he's going to *drive* from Toronto to Vancouver to pick me up. He'll arrive in about three days, and we'll go home. I somehow manage to talk him out of it.

Sometimes, as I'm lying in this bed, I get visitors. I know this happens but it's blurry and weirdly intangible. Blair's still got the phone book typing job so he's working long hours but comes in late in the evenings.

My dog, Susie, is at home; Maia and Colin help Blair take care of her and come in and visit when they can. My friend Adrian comes at some point. He brings books and magazines, and we walk around the ward. We end up in a garden courtyard in the middle of the floor. It's surreal and unexpected, a calm in the middle of the chaos. I have a vague fantasy as we sit and breathe in the plants that I'm a Buddhist in a monastery, and my tie-up gown and pants are my spiritual robes.

It is said that the body has no memory of pain. I don't know quite where I first heard this—I believe in relation to childbirth—the idea being that if anyone truly remembered, no one would ever have more than one child. When I ask my friend Ethan about this, he says, "We didn't really talk about pain in those terms in medical school at all. Unfortunately, it's all about neuroreceptors and the most mechanical, cold understanding of the chemical reactions we perceive as pain. But not about what it really means to feel it."

But I remember every detail of every ravaging, injurious invasion into my body. And in these moments of pain, I find it impossible to conjure even the simplest memory of pleasure. The vague relief that comes when the pain is taken away is too tainted by the swollen aftertaste of violation to cause any joy. Hospital is the forced abandonment of control—the violent, bloody, yet sterile bruising of flesh. The taste of the hospital lingers. I can be anywhere, doing anything, and the poisonous taste of laxatives for bowel prep can make my jaw tense and shake until my whole body feels paralyzed. I can remember the smell of the boiled plastic euphemistically described as food that arrived at the side of my bed after I spent the day retching, and the voice of the doctor—"Make sure you eat; you won't get better if you don't eat" —with the scolding undertone. What were once indulgent sensual pleasures—the joys of tastes and the freedom of nudity—are robbed and coerced.

The best way to describe a hospital experience is a clenching of the chest. A flinching at the constant incursions of my bodily boundaries, a sudden intake of breath to prevent myself from lashing out. There's a perpetual nausea that lives in my nasal cavities as I refuse to really look at myself or where I am because if I do, I start to shake. Sometimes with uncontrollable vigour, and the tears start. I have a repetitive thought that arises when I revisit these moments that goes something like this: *It wasn't really that bad; you're totally exaggerating.* I think that voice is the piece of myself who gets me through — the stiff upper lip and ram-rod-straight-spined version of Julie who smiles and laughs and charms her way to the other side of the trauma. So I hold these thoughts, this pain, burrowed deeply in the only spot that's still mine — the pinpoint at the dead centre between my brows — the dot where resistance still lives.

When I finally get discharged, I go home and fill my prescription for oral steroids. I take the dose and then, within the hour, have cramps so severe that I think I'm going to vomit. The world is spinning, and my gut is convinced that I've actually been drinking the acid from a giant battery. I sit up in my bed, trying to wait out the nausea until the Gravol kicks in with some relief. The torment isn't so much the pain, as brutal as it is, but this fear that if I throw up the steroids, my adrenal glands will shut down. An extreme and paranoid sort of understanding of what I was told, but it haunts me nonetheless.

Corticosteroids are a powerful medication that increases the cortisol in the body, a substance naturally produced by the adrenal glands. When you take more than your body would naturally produce, your adrenal glands stop functioning. For this reason, as soon as you go on them, you're emphatically told that you cannot suddenly stop taking them. I'm scared that violently vomiting up my first oral dose is sufficient reason to go back into the hospital. When my stomach finally settles down, I fall asleep, only to be woken up hourly with a bladder more full and active than it's ever been in my entire life. I've never peed so much before. I start worrying that something's amiss with my kidney function and phone my floor of the hospital the next day to see if the doctor who supervised my care is available. He's on a two-week vacation. They offer to page the resident who's been taking care of me. She phones me back and says that she doesn't know why I'm passing so much urine. She doesn't sound very concerned but suggests that I go back to emerg. I figure she's just saying that as a default professional version of "I have no idea." I wait it out and the peeing subsides.

Looking back, as I edit this with the wisdom of many more hospitalizations behind me, I can see pretty clearly that it's the bags and bags of saline solution they pumped into my veins to hydrate me that was gushing out of my bladder upon discharge, but no one told me. Being sick turns out to be a crash course in learning how to live with myself. Not hiding in the frazzled busyness of day-to-day life but constantly engaging with and often interrogating myself. *Who am I? Why am I here? What do I really want to be doing with my time?*

I hear the refrain over and over again from people going through the dark places of illness who now phone or email me for advice. "I just want to get back to work, get on with my life, that's all I want" — as if there's some inherent virtue in working. And, of course, there's nothing wrong with wanting to creatively interact with the world and participate. But illness isn't an exception to life. It's not some kind of stepping out period where life *stops.* It's not even a pause or a break. It's the most challenging internal work I've ever done.

I see now how I always blame myself: *I wouldn't have gotten sick if only I had ... or hadn't ... or realized ... been stronger ... smarter ... better.* The guilt is pervasive and often stoked by people in authority, but it is also the only control I have in the moment. If I maintain the staunch belief that I started this, then maybe it's not spiralling outside of my control; maybe, the logical subplot is that I can stop it. Power in guilt. The crucial difference between the fictions I cultivate about myself and the truths I discover is impact. Sometimes fiction is more appealing.

2. Home

You don't need to be helped any longer. You've always had
the power to go back to Kansas.

> — Glinda the Good Witch talking to Dorothy,
> *The Wizard of Oz*

The second night home is the most peaceful of my life.

Lying in my bed with Blair on one side and my dog, Susie, on the other.
No nurses, no wavering vitals, no roommates trying to crawl into my bed.
When I wake up, I feel more calm and serene than I have ever felt. I book
my flight back to Toronto and see only a couple of people before I leave.
It's a strange way to move back home. Blair stays in Vancouver to pack
up our apartment with Maia and Colin, while I fly home with Susie. The
three of them are following in a few weeks. I tell the agent when I book
my ticket that I need assistance through the airport. You're supposed to
ask the staff as you go through the gate, but I'm too embarrassed. Even
though I'm still extremely weak, I'm afraid that people will think I'm
faking it — exaggerating to get attention — or, worse yet, that I'm actually
ill and someone to be pitied. So, with a heavy backpack on my back and
my dog in her carrier on my front, I drag myself through departures in
Vancouver and past security, where carts are no longer allowed. The plane

ride is boring, nondescript, with the occasional interruption of Susie's chin in my hands after I illicitly unzip her carrier.

I've never been so relieved to see anyone as I am to see my mum waiting for me at the Toronto airport. She looks thinner than I've ever seen her, drained by worry, and it scares me. I feel irrationally responsible for creating this fragility in my mother.

It's a beautiful summer in Toronto, so I spend a lot of time with Susie outside. I visit with friends and soak up some sun. The steroids are now fully working, making digestion easy and my appetite soar. I have energy. Blair returns and we settle into creating a life in Toronto. It's an awkward transition for me. Despite all the issues of living in Vancouver, I did get used to having my own adult space. Living with my parents again definitely feels like a step backwards. For one thing, Maia, Colin, Blair, and I were always very flexible about food. Sharing, cooking, shopping at whatever hours and in whatever ways we felt like at the time. Our kitchen wasn't big enough for a table, so we ate on the couches in the main room.

With my parents, preparing and eating food is carried out with military precision. For example, my sister, Joanne, and I often laugh about having to declare our banana intake in advance. Bananas sit in the basement cold cellar at a specific shade of yellow with a hint of green. When they are brought into the warmth of the kitchen, they're perfectly yellow about twelve hours later, and maintain that ideal hue for another twelve hours before browning. So in the evening, my dad asks who wants a banana the next day. Over the course of the following day, you must eat your banana. And never, God forbid, eat two, as Blair innocently did once. When we first started dating in 1998, I mentioned something to Blair about Susie liking bananas. He found this ridiculous and handed her one, thinking she wouldn't want it. My twelve-pound schnauzer took the entire banana, skin and all, and ran away like she'd won the jackpot. Horrified, I chased her down to where my dad was watching TV. Thankfully he was too engrossed in the program to see me prying the now-tooth-marked banana out of her mouth. Despite the fact that, years later, this is a story we all share and find funny, the underlying seriousness of such matters hasn't really shifted.

Everyone sits at the table to eat dinner at exactly 5:30 p.m. every evening. If you're not home, your dinner will be left in the oven or on the stove, waiting to be reheated. There's an intuitive understanding and shared code about exactly how much food and what kind of balance of food one should take. For example, don't eat *all* the meat or *all* the rice, leaving only vegetables for leftovers. I wasn't aware of the precision of our family's food code until I painstakingly explained it to Blair and he laughed — thinking I couldn't possibly be serious — and I had to stress to him how very serious it was. Dinnertime is also where all the most heated arguments about the world, the family, school, work, and politics happen. The more wine that is consumed, the louder it gets. I was never aware of this dynamic until Blair was sitting next to me, and I occasionally heard him squeak or start the first half of a word in the middle of conversations. This would happen repeatedly until I raised my voice and emphatically put my hands out saying, "Shhh! Everyone be quiet. Blair's trying to say something." And we'd all get very, very quiet so he could contribute.

Although my dad grew up in the north of England, his background is Irish. My mum was born in an Italian mountain village where her family goes back further than history even records. Growing up, when people asked what my cultural background was, I explained that, although I was born in England, I'm Irish Italian. People almost universally reacted the same way. "Wow! That's intense," or "You must have a really bad temper," or "That's two passionate groups of people!" or "So I guess you're *really* Catholic." I always laughed along, kind of agreeing and kind of thinking they were exaggerating. But cultural stereotypes aside, I can say without question that my family can be very loud. Now, back after a year of bowel distress, I start to feel acutely in my body how this lively atmosphere is not particularly conducive to me calmly and easily digesting my food.

Soon after returning, I have an appointment with Dr. Lane, my specialist. We figure out a schedule for tapering the oral steroids. It will be several months before I can come off completely. I can't sleep much from steroid-insomnia. I see my family doctor and tell him the only time I can sleep is when I take Gravol. He cautiously prescribes me something to help. Another impact from the steroids is that my cheeks are so round people I don't know speak to me as if I am a child. I'm quite short anyway and don't necessarily dress like a grown-up, so the round face erases whatever superficial status I attained by becoming an adult.

I remember going to pick up my medication and wondering if I really did look fourteen. "You have to write out the instructions really clearly or she won't understand what to do," the pharmacist says, exasperated when the assistant complains that the tapering instructions for the steroids won't fit on the label.

"I know how to take my medication." I cut in loudly from the other side of the counter. "I understand."

The pharmacist completely ignores me and comes over to tell my mother to buy me a calendar; otherwise, I'm sure to get confused and misunderstand what to take when. I intervene once more, firmly assuring him that I know what I'm doing. He finally surrenders the medication. To my mother.

Giant mood swings are typical when taking steroids. Pills, pills, and more pills leave me in pharmaceutical haze. And I'm sure the trauma doesn't help. Cheer by sheer force of will is my new method. I can taste the pain, the disappointment, the fear. I remember driving through an industrial area near my house and thinking myself into being happy —swallowing up all the letdown of having to drop everything and telling myself that I'm okay. This is all for the best. Then it occurs to me that instead of blocking all the pain, I might as well indulge in it. Let it wash through my senses as if it's something exquisite, overpowering in its taste. Like liquid white chocolate.

I make sure to keep my life busy. I swim, read novels, and enrol in a

French class. I join the gym. I find that intense physical activity gives me enough of a buzz to subdue my occasional evening bouts of psychotic rage—another pleasant side effect of steroids. It's funny how I can be very expressive of some things but be absolutely devoid of the tools to express others. I just get this very tense and hyperactive sort of anger surging through me, and I don't know what to do, what to say, or how to get any relief. The other end of this hyperactivity is extreme clarity. I come up with very clear and detailed visions of academic work I can pursue and specific ways of finishing my degree from Toronto.

My supervisor, Tara, agrees to do courses by distance with me, including my thesis, and agrees with the courses I want to take in Toronto. I make several proposals to the department, but they insist that there's a residency requirement. If I want to take courses in Toronto, that's fine, but I have to return to Vancouver in a year to finish. At this point, I can't see how I can possibly commit to living in Vancouver for another eight-month period, even in a year's time. The final straw is when I write an extensive proposal outlining how I want to proceed with my program and nobody responds. It's summertime and I understand that people might not be there, so a week later, I phone the department, and the secretary says she'll see if the director is available. The secretary returns to me on the phone, long distance from Toronto.

"The answer is no," she says.

I'm shocked. "Excuse me, did she give any explanation? Can I expect to hear why?"

"That's what she said: the answer is no."

And she hangs up. Snot-Face doesn't even bother to respond to my email or deign to speak to me herself. Just a cryptic denial through her secretary. Leaving me, four thousand kilometres away, completely broken. I feel like I have no option but to take a medical withdrawal. I've paid tuition for the summer term for the reading course I ended up being too sick to actually complete while still in Vancouver. In some weird bureaucratic detail, because "leaves" aren't granted retroactively I can only get my summer tuition back by withdrawing entirely from my program, retroactively to the end of April. I submit the medical documentation the university demands, and my withdrawal is finalized. Tara is supportive. She tells me just to take care of my health. "Everything will be there for you when you're feeling better."

I'm feeling frustrated and antsy. I want to get on with my master's degree; my life has been disrupted enough. I make an appointment at the university near my parents' home where I did my undergraduate degree. It's too late to actually get into the master's program, and there's apparently no such thing as a transfer in grad school. The director of the program I'm interested in is happy to allow me to take courses as a visiting student but wonders why I won't just finish the degree I've already started in Vancouver, from a distance.

"We have a student doing the same thing right now. She had some personal reasons why she had to return, actually to Vancouver. So she's taking some courses there, writing her thesis from there, and she'll still get her degree from us."

"I don't really understand why," I tell her. "But they won't let me do that. They have some kind of residency requirement."

So I enrol in some graduate courses and get part-time work doing some student organizing. Through September, things are pretty good. It's comforting to be in familiar environments as I'm healing my body. My good friend Dawn is starting grad school at the same university in Toronto. She has very recently given birth to an amazing little boy, and we take a class together with her thesis supervisor, who has enthusiastically invited Dawn and her breastfeeding newborn into the seminar. Blair and I continue living with my parents; there's just no way we can risk getting our own place with my health being so unstable. Blair decides to take on a trade. He's always enjoyed working with his hands and prefers to spend his days physically active. My dad is a carpenter and provides all the necessary support and information to get Blair started in a carpenters' apprenticeship program. His employment is steady, and it's a lot more interesting than typing the phone book. And although it's not exactly in the field of his visual arts degree, the classes, at least, engage his considerable visual acuity and let him use his talents and dexterity for fine detail.

Every week, I reduce the steroids as scheduled, and every week, I have less energy and feel slightly more ill. This is typical with steroid withdrawal, so I just wait for my body to pick up the slack, gently encouraging it. "Colon, heal thyself!"

Any impact makes me bleed more. I can't do much at the gym anymore. I feel the judgmental eyes of the older women bearing into me when physical activity becomes a struggle, as if I just wasn't trying. The sort of smug self-satisfaction that they're more fit than a woman twenty years their junior. One woman openly criticizes me for going slower than her on the treadmill; another shouts after me when I rushed out of a step class to get to the toilet, "Don't give up now!" I fantasize about designing a T-shirt that outlines my diagnosis and current symptoms with a giant middle finger that lights up when activated by the heat of a self-righteous stare.

3. Me and Charles Darwin

Years later, when I'm doing my chronic illness research, I read that Charles Darwin was sick most of his adult life.

At the time, this is a marginal detail in his biography. He did his research and writing mostly between the bed and the bath. Why couldn't I finish *my* graduate studies from there? Why couldn't I earn money by researching and writing in bed? What is it about the world today that defines us by our bodily health, and why are the ways and form in which we are allowed to participate so incredibly regimented?

When I initially started having bloody movements again, Dr. Lane prescribed the anti-inflammatory medication I was on in enema form. So now, every night, I have to lie on my side and pump my rectum and colon full of cold liquid medication. I immediately have to roll onto my stomach to make sure I retain it for the night. The impulse to release the fluid when cramping and spasming from the cold is intense.

As I lie like this, I urge Blair, "Talk to me, tell me a story, anything. Distract me."

The pain usually passes within about ten minutes and I can go to sleep.

When this method still doesn't relieve my symptoms, my doctor increases the dose to two enemas a day—an anti-inflammatory enema at night, a steroid enema in the morning. I try working and doing the morning enemas for a while. It means setting the clock for 5:30 a.m., doing the enema, and lying perfectly still for at least an hour, because as soon as I move, I can't hold it any longer, and I have to rush to the toilet and let it gush out. I watch episodes of *Buffy the Vampire Slayer* to distract myself from the pain. Joanne kindly bought me videotapes. Fictional kicks, punches, slaying, and witty repartee are my only escape.

At this point, Dr. Lane starts talking about "other options." If we can't control the disease with these medications, then I have to consider either trying more potent medications that modulate my immune system or having my colon removed surgically. My symptoms continue to rage. The more I try to taper off with lower doses of steroids, the more my body rebels. I continue going to work. One day, I find myself rushing into a washroom after making an announcement to a large lecture hall. If there hadn't been a toilet right there, I never would have made it. It's a matter of seconds. I see blood filling the toilet bowl, and in this moment, some part of me knows definitively that I will need the surgery. Some might call it defeatism; I call it realistic knowledge that I somehow manage to suppress anyway. I go into the hall and resume the conversation I'm having with my co-worker. I feel a weird sense of detachment, numbness. He's someone I've known for years but never particularly gotten along with. So we've been bickering all day—about everything from minute details about the materials we're using and direction we're walking to bigger fights about political choices each of us have made over the previous few years. My fear and distress is just too profound and overwhelming to reveal myself in any way at all to this colleague.

Classes become increasingly difficult to attend, and much to my embarrassment, I have to leave early-morning messages at work saying that I can't come in. I hate having to go back on things I promised to do. I'm also very nervous that people won't believe me after my Vancouver experiences. Thankfully, there's a world of difference. Everyone is incredibly understanding. Both of my professors at school insist that I just concentrate on getting well: no pressure, no stress. My work colleagues feel terrible.

"Oh my God, did we make you sick again?"

"Have we been working you too hard?"

"What if you just had to sit behind a table and not do any running around?"

And this certainly helps. Sitting behind tables on quieter campuses with friendly faces and nearby toilets accommodates a lot of my physical symptoms and allows me to work.

As the number of my bowel movements and the amount of blood in them increases every day, the enemas become increasingly painful and difficult to retain. My specialist gets me an appointment with a surgeon and a prescription for an immune-suppressive drug. She calls me on the phone to explain how to take the medication. We'll start slowly and work up to the full dose within a month. At this point, it will take three months before we know with any certainty if the medication is working. I have to continue the enemas twice a day. She's concerned about the long-term side effects of the steroids on my body.

"You already have the moon face," she sensitively comments.

She hasn't seen me for more than a month at this point, and has a full load of patients. I am horrified that she remembers the size of the ever-expanding mass that has become my face. She gives me the anti-liability lecture about all the rare side effects that can be caused by the drug. Lymphoma is the one that sticks in my mind. My sister received an email a few months earlier about a well-known professor in her field who had died in hospital from complications of ulcerative colitis. Further probing revealed that it was actually an experimental immune-modulator drug that she was receiving intravenously that had killed her.

My mum picks up the prescription and brings it home. I look at the greenish-yellow pills. They're ridged and shaped like figure eights with a flat centre. All I can think of is cancer in my lymph nodes, Hodgkin's disease. My cousin had Hodgkin's disease in his late twenties. I look at the pills and imagine putting cancer in my mouth and down my throat with a quick swig of water. I can't do it. I have such a skill for demonstrating all the rare side effects from my disease, why not from the medication?

At this point, my day looks like this:

Wake up, do steroid enema. Take antacid pill to reverse the acid reflux caused by steroids.

Breakfast. Take steroids. Take bowel anti-inflammatory. Take calcium and vitamin D to help control the potential bone loss caused by steroids.

Lunch. Take more bowel anti-inflammatory.

Dinner. More bowel anti-inflammatory. Another antacid pill. Take iron.

Bedtime. Final dose of bowel anti-inflammatory and then the second enema. In addition, anti-nauseant pills, sleeping pills, and Tylenol, as needed.

When all this isn't working, there's just no way I can attend any classes or go out and work. Surgery starts to feel more and more inevitable. The thought terrifies me, but being permanently on medication that can cause infertility and cancer seems even less appealing than the knife. I want an outside perspective.

I send my uncle an email with the subject line "the fix it or nix it debate." Uncle Tony is Mum's younger brother, a progressive-minded writer who lives with his wife in an apartment downtown. After we first moved from England, when I was six, I used to phone him a few times a week just to chat. No matter how busy he was, he always called me back and always had something to say that I would unquestioningly accept as truth. A couple of years earlier, he'd had a serious stomach ulcer that needed to be operated on, and I want to know what he thinks.

He phones me and warns me about my upcoming appointment with the surgeon.

"Remember," he says, "surgeons cut; it's what they do. Make sure you've explored every option before you let him talk you into it. See as many specialists as you can. Don't do this except as your last resort."

I look into all the experimental drugs that are being tested. Dr. Lane has the people running a clinical trial phone me. This medication they're studying is leading the way for genetically engineered medications. It actually has mouse DNA in it, which I find somewhat off-putting, but it has proven very effective in rheumatoid arthritis, another inflammatory autoimmune disease. The medication can only be administered by infusion. I find various websites for class action suits against the pharmaceutical company that manufactures the drug. Apparently, some people went into cardiac arrest and died while going through the infusions. My mind immediately skips back to my thirty-eight-beats-a-minute heart rate that no one in the hospital really managed to explain. It turns out that I'm not eligible for the trial anyway because I'm too sick. I joke that I don't want to grow fur and develop a squeak instead of a voice anyway. I do an excellent mouse impression.

4. Remember This Scene

So I go and meet George Singer, surgeon. His briefcase is battered and his secretary calls him George. He has an open and warm face and seems genuinely sympathetic. He takes me into the examining room and leaves while I change into the gown. He comes back and asks me to roll onto my side.

"What are you going to do?" I ask.

I'm lying, covered with a thin sheet, on a cold slab of metal. I'm up to twelve bowel movements a day at this point. *Raw* and *inflamed* are only words and, as such, do not adequately cover the pain and discomfort I am in. I barely slept at all the night before, and as a result, I'm extremely nauseated. This is a repeating theme. On the drive home, I scrawl a description into my notebook—a set of instructions aimed at the surgeon himself to try to make him understand the physicality of this bodily experience:

> So here's an exercise. Put your hand on the very front of
> your collarbone. The two bumps in the centre of your chest
> at the base of your throat. Imagine someone has tied a string
> around the passageways directly above and behind this bone.
> Those you use for eating, drinking, breathing. The strings

are attached to strings coming from the back of your nasal cavities and throat and are being pulled down into your gut. Your rectum and the area just on the inside of each hip feel sore, aching and expanded, like a weight. The strings have pulled these areas up and have become tangled. Every time you move you are at risk of retching and spasming. All of these movements are caught up with one another. You are weak, tired, shaky, and dizzy.

He shows me this instrument: a small, hand-held scope.

"I'm just going to take a look," he says.

First, he shoves his giant, sausage finger into my rectum.

I tell him, "That really, really hurts. You're really, really hurting me."

He ignores me and proceeds to put his little toy up inside of me.

"This will just be uncomfortable for a minute," he assures me. I don't feel assured.

When I tell my friend Ali (who you'll meet very soon) this story, she says, "He's like Jacques Cartier! Brave explorer looking for treasure with his telescope..." It's too perfect an analogy.

He fits in with the colonization allegory with surgical precision as he proclaims triumphantly, "Yup, you definitely have ulcerative colitis."

Give the man a bloody medal. We never could have established that from my chart. We go back into his office, where we discuss the surgical options. He agrees that if my disease cannot be controlled by the enemas and I can't come off the steroids, it's a valid choice for me to opt for the surgery rather than take the immune-modulator. He takes my email address and offers to send me links to illustrated websites describing the surgery in detail. I explain how painful and difficult it is for me to retain the enemas and describe how many excruciating bowel movements I am having a day. Dr. Singer asks me, "So what do you do?"

I look at him blankly, not quite sure what he means.

"What's your job? Are you in school?"

I'm frustrated. "When I'm well, I'm a graduate student. I do research work and get jobs doing political organizing. But right now, this, this is what I do. I don't 'do' anything."

It's at moments like that that I feel the most disconnected. If the surgeon doesn't get it, when he's talking about hacking my colon out, then who does get it? Who actually understands the minute-to-minute agony? I go into the hallway and book an appointment for a scope. Once he's given me a colonoscopy, we can discuss a date for the surgery.

Medical professionals place patients on tables to be examined, mapped out, dissected, and repaired. And while, in the abstract, I appreciate that this activity can lead to brilliant cures, it makes me feel like a slab of meat; as if my entering the doctor's office and getting on his table means that he owns my body somehow. My desire to turn this moment into an opportunity to teach manners to med students starts to swell. I tell myself that if they just *understood* and could somehow personally experience the feelings in my body in their own bodies, even just in their imaginations, then they would never behave so inappropriately again. I will get the opportunity to use this moment, this piece of writing, to educate health care professionals in the years, and chapters, to come.

5. Civil War

The following week, Maia's mum dies.

First, there's the funeral home. Then the mass, the wake, the burial. I want to be there for all of it, so I am. I manage for these short spurts to be well enough to function, even slightly energized. The time is so terrible for Maia that my concerns about being well enough just fade into the background of my consciousness, and my body complies with several days of moderate health and vitality.

My condition spirals downwards. Dr. Lane starts giving me weekly appointments on her office day before any of her scheduled patients arrive. I hear her office administrator telling another doctor's office that the regular waiting time for appointments is about six months. She puts me back on the steroids, this time with a dose that's actually double the dose I was on when I got out of hospital last time. She thinks this is our only hope of getting the symptoms under control. Except this time the symptoms just keep getting worse. People in my family come and go, continuing with their daily activities. They go out at night. Socialize.

I lie in bed. Trying to retain enemas. Trying to keep some kind of bowel control. Whenever I do venture out, I'm constantly aware that I may need to rush and find a washroom. I'm tired and unhappy. I'm entirely dependent on Blair and my family for everything. Money, entertainment, comfort. And I start to notice a theme — that since I've become ill, people keep telling me how lucky I am to have Blair. It's not so much the sentiment I object to; it's the fact that no one has ever said this before. Now I'm suddenly undeserving of love — damaged goods, broken, a "lemon." My illness has devalued me to such an extent that our relationship is no longer something that we mutually built and developed, it's something that *I* have lucked into.

When I tell Dr. Lane that I'm not feeling any better, she says, "You should *not* be having these symptoms on sixty milligrams of steroids."

To put this in perspective, I should explain that the body naturally produces the equivalent of about five to ten milligrams of steroids as a natural hormone called cortisol. In a healthy body, this is generally enough to suppress inflammatory responses, and if it's not, the adrenal glands will produce more. Twelve times that amount taken artificially should therefore have some impact on inflammation. She's unequivocal.

"You need to go into the hospital and get your medication intravenously."

So it's November 30, 2002. I am back in the emerg at my parents' local hospital. I am lying flat on my back on a gurney. Face to face with the arrogant, self-important Dr. Cartwright.

"Go home. Your specialist should be treating this from home. What do you want me to do?"

The irony of being asked this in an ER for the second time in six months does not escape me. The easiest way to get on a doctor's bad side is to tell him what to do. It is, without a doubt, a rhetorical question. But at the same time, it's a question that opens the door to patients like me telling stubborn medical professionals *exactly* what we want them to do.

"I would like you to follow my specialist's instructions and put me on Solu-Medrol steroid IV."

Predictably, this annoys him supremely.

"Well, you can stay until I get your blood results."

He lets out a great sigh and hurries out in search of a new patient to harass. *I can stay? How generous.*

Melisse, the nurse, comes in next. She actually took my blood earlier, admiring my high pain tolerance as she poked around for a vein to start my IV.

She leans in now to tell me that she's already seen my blood results.

"Your white count is way too high; there's no way he can send you home."

Evidently, she's been listening to my conversations with Cartwright and has similar feelings about his bedside manner. In fact, she probably dislikes him far more than I do, seeing as she's actually working with him and his intense arrogance.

He comes back and reluctantly grunts at me that he'll start the Solu-Medrol steroid IV.

It helps when I mention that I'm also under the care of Dr. Singer, head of the hospital's surgery department. I feel like I need to make a bit of a case for Dr. Singer, the surgeon, here. I'm aware that in the writing of the Jacques Cartier incident, he comes across pretty badly. But, in his defence, he's old school, just following his training. In his mind, his methods are the best ones to create remissions and cures in patients. As a human, he's extremely kind, and as a surgeon, he's very well reputed. He comes to visit me, completely unnecessarily, in the middle of his busy surgeon's schedule.

He jokes as I lie for the second time in a row on a gurney in the middle of the ER. "I see we've got you in the luxury suite."

He supports my decision to choose surgery over trying new medications, if I can't stabilize coming off of the steroids. He feels this is a valid choice. One could argue that it's his third, invisible eye (dubbed by a friend as "Scalpel Eye") that has given him this insight into patient rights. The eye hovers almost imperceptibly in the centre of his forehead, focused intently on my rebel colon. In my uncle's ominous words, "Surgeons cut; it's what they do." But, at least, he's making me feel that I'm entitled to make a decision.

Dr. Lane isn't working this weekend, so I'm introduced to a new specialist, Dr. Bird. He decides to schedule a scope for two days later, so I have to start the prep in the emergency room. Dr. Bird demands to know why I haven't started the immune-modulator drug. I explain that I'm concerned about the side effects, and skeptical about whether it will work anyway, and have decided that I'd rather have surgery than permanently take this medication.

He looks at me with undisguised impatience. "No," he says, "you don't need surgery. Take the immune-modulator. It will get you off of the steroids and you'll be fine."

I'm taken aback, but not exactly in a position to argue. It's easy for him to so casually commit the rest of my life to taking a medication that can cause cancer and infertility.

There is an irreconcilable distance between what is institutionally taught as good practice and what I perceive as a patient. Doctors are taught to question everything: past diagnoses, patients' accounts of symptoms and history. Thoroughness in theory means challenging the accuracy of every detail to establish the soundest analysis. Each doctor is taught to greet me as a fresh case, holding no prejudice. Many doctors in my experience use this as an excuse to be bullies. And even when it's done "right," the only way I process the perpetual questioning when I'm feeling unbearably ill is to feel cross-examined, interrogated, challenged, and not believed.

Still in the emergency ward, I am given my first dose of poisonous-tasting bowel prep to clean my bowel of all its contents. Drinking this laxative induces urgent bouts of diarrhea. This is predictably unpleasant in an emerg with two shared washrooms for the entire ward.

I am finally taken to a room—511, Bed 1. By now, the intravenous steroids are definitely working, and I'm feeling a lot better. Dr. Bird comes to see me again, and tells me that I won't be discharged until my white blood count is a lot lower. This count goes up when the body is responding to inflammation or infection.

A very pleasant woman called Paula is in Bed 2, in recovery from breast cancer. Her chemotherapy went well in terms of beating the cancer cells, but it's now wreaking havoc with her healthy cells. Her white count is far too low, leaving her prone to infections, fevers, and chills. She's not allowed to leave until it has risen sufficiently. She really wants to be out for the weekend because her daughter is having an engagement party.

We joke that a simple blood transfusion can solve both of our problems—with a little mix and match, we can end up somewhere in the healthy middle. We tell one of the nurses. She doesn't laugh. Instead, looking horrified, she asks perfectly seriously, "Am I going to have to watch this room?"

Right at the time of this hospitalization, the Ontario government launches an advertising campaign about the wonders they've done for the health care system. They have a nurse pledging her undying support of Conservative Premier Ernie Eves and his government. When the commercial comes on, I feel like I'm lying in the middle of a George Orwell novel, hearing the cheery political health care commentary in the backdrop while the nurses constantly rush from one medical crisis to the next. A nurse is in the room one time when the commercial comes on. She immediately starts shouting foul things at the TV, and I gleefully egg her on.

Tuesday morning arrives: scope day.

It's an entirely different specialist who's set to do it, but Dr. Lane assures me that I'll like him.

The first thing I remember him saying to me is "Guess what my record is, how many scopes I've performed in one day?"

As I lie there, terrified, I smile and say flippantly, "Oh, I don't know. A thousand?"

"No," he says, annoyed, deflated, the wind knocked out of his sails. "Forty! That's a lot, you know."

And he's right; it *is* a lot. Ethan tells me later that doctors bill two hundred dollars a scope. "That's eight grand!" Ethan exclaims. For just one day of inflicting torturous scopes.

But, somehow, this time, it doesn't hurt very much. It quickly becomes evident why.

"You're clear. There's hardly any disease here at all. Look at the healthy pink tissue!"

Dr. 40-Scope writes in my chart (which I read on the way back up to my room) that I have only very mild distal disease. He says that it can be treated by enemas, that I certainly don't need surgery, and that if I should flare up again coming off of the steroids, then I should be medicated with the immune-modulator.

There seems to be a consensus building that if I can't get off of the steroids this time, this immune-modulator drug is my future. Consensus among collaborating doctors. Collaborators against consent.

The consistency with which doctors in hospitals from coast to coast treat me is beginning to make me paranoid. I wonder if there's something about *me* that makes them all feel like my spirit has to be crushed before they can get on with their important business. But now I understand from watching friends of mine go through medical school that it's really not me. It is all of them. The militarism that is medical training: social isolation, sleep deprivation, highly stressful environment. When they are weak and almost broken, tell them they are God. Or, at least, soldiers in the Army of Life and Death. The system creates a profound sense of entitlement in doctors. "We have worked so hard, withstood so much. Just to help *you*. Because we *love* medicine. Are *you* deserving?" There is so much pressure on doctors to be "right" and so much competition in medical training that it can produce a vicious response to feelings of impotence and ignorance.

This poses a particular problem for me, with my autoimmune condition

that defies expected outcomes and fluctuates so wildly between manage-
ability and chaos. The attitudinal difference between doctors who have
actual immediate knowledge or experience with my disease compared to
those who don't is phenomenal. At this point, the only time I have been
admitted to a hospital in a way that wasn't completely dehumanizing was
in the downtown ER in Vancouver, when the doctor had a cousin with my
condition. So far, it seems like doctors who manage to keep their humanity
do it *despite* their training. No one knows what started this civil war in my
body—my immune system's repeated attacks on my colon, my skin and
my joints. And now I am forced to engage in civil wars with doctors in
order to treat it.

6. New Year's is for Chumps

Dr. Lane comes to see me in my hospital room. She explains that I can taper quickly off the oral steroids and that the enemas should clear up the remainder of my disease. She explains that the intravenous steroids can be extremely effective in healing disease. She's pleased. I'm elated. Dr. Lane is someone who somehow manages to balance scientific intelligence with sensitivity. She ends most of our appointments with the words "because I want you to be well."

I tell her about my run-in with Cartwright, the emerg doctor who didn't want to admit me. First, she explains that there is no way for her to have me directly admitted. The way the hospital system is set up means that patients have to be assessed through the emergency department. This is the process I learn about years later in the health policy lecture on how chronically ill patients become bed-blockers.

Then she tells me, "Julie, you have a serious, chronic illness. Any time you feel sick enough, you should be admitted to the hospital."

I am comforted by the vindication but despaired by the prognosis.

I get more books on food and digestion, including one promising natural relief for colitis symptoms through diet. I am determined that I am going to maintain this remission. I set out to find a naturopath. I want all the possible answers I can find.

I remember walking into the naturopath's office and just feeling so tired. I want some control. She seems sympathetic. I fill out a massive questionnaire in her lobby. My entire life history, every injury I've ever sustained, and every medication and morsel of food that has ever passed my lips. The naturopath (let's call her Frances) hooks me up to electronic sensors that are supposed to detect food sensitivities and areas of "stress" in my body. Blair thinks the whole thing is cracked. I feel like a desperate sinner, looking for salvation from the only source bold enough to promise it. I'm supposed to keep my hands still while her machines process my sensitivity, but she keeps asking me questions, and I explain that I'm Italian and my hands just can't help moving while I talk. She asks me if I've been experiencing low moods. I find the question a bit odd after I've just described my year. Frances assures me that once I've eliminated gluten and anything that has ever been in any way processed and start taking the ten thousand vitamins and supplements she's prescribing, my "low moods" will be no more.

She doesn't seem to have any sympathy for what I've been through at all. I get the impression that she's just never had any kind of health issue in her life.

"So you eat a lot of bread and pasta." Frances states this as a fact, and I wonder if her machine's just told her this.

"Not that much. Why?"

"Well," she says confidently, "you said you're Italian."

"Half," I answer. "My dad's not Italian, and he does most of the cooking. He never cooks pasta."

Frances doesn't seem put out that her assumption is so far off. She goes on to explain in a really patronizing tone that our culture sees food as something to comfort, entertain, and socialize with, instead of just nourishment to fuel our bodies. I just have to stop seeing it like that. I tell her that I'm not doing anything until I put it past my specialist.

Dr. Lane is extremely irritated with the idea that a colitis patient would be put on a restrictive diet. The biggest nutritional risk for me, in her opinion, is malnutrition caused from a decreased appetite and fear that eating will make my symptoms worse. Taking away all of my staple foods at once is not a strategy likely to lead to wellness. She doesn't have anything to worry about on my behalf. I last about thirty-six hours on the naturopath diet.

The diet sheets Frances gives me are really strict regimens with exact times I need to eat exact types of food. Everything on the allowable food lists is boiled, baked, and generally taste-free. The bottom line is that I don't feel any kind of support from her at all. Her sanctimonious approach makes me feel like she's blaming me for being sick or, at the very least, totally unconscious that her words about my food choices could be taken that way. Nothing in the history of the universe has ever tasted as good as that chicken in spinach-wrap pita with creamy dressing I eat to break the Frances-induced fast. My mood is instantly elevated by the outlawed tastes. I stop taking the remedies and supplements when I can't sleep because my hands are tingling and itching so badly.

I start trying to reorganize my life. I've missed so much class that I have no idea how I'm going to get the credits for the courses I'm enrolled in. But both of my professors agree to let me write one final paper for each of them to make up for the rest of my mark. I expect to finish both of my papers by mid-January. But the quick tapering off from the steroids wreaks havoc with my energy level and concentration. This is supposed to pass. I go for a bone-density scan. It shows mild bone loss — osteopenia. With exercise, "weight-bearing" activity, and calcium and vitamin D, I can undo the steroids' effect on my weakening bones.

I'm still really tired, but I know that this is a normal effect of steroid withdrawal. Christmas is nice. New Year's less so. New Year's Eve has always been my least favourite holiday. It could be because I hate anticipation of any sort. There's always too much build-up. Or it could be because I'm cursed. New Year's Eve 2002, I begin my next flare-up. Always highly skilled in the art of denial, I decide that it's the flu. I tell Dr. Lane my theory. She gives me The Look but, to her credit, entertains the idea.

"Well, colitis patients are definitely more prone to catch these things. And it would be a lot harder for you to get over…"

As the flare-up continues, I'm convinced that it will just solve itself. *Because I'm not sick anymore. The camera has seen my colon, and it is not diseased. This is just mild distal disease, in my rectum, causing bleeding. The diarrhea is from the flu. Now it's from my period. It's going to go away.* I am entirely dependent on large amounts of meaningful human contact. I need to bounce off people constantly, feed from their ideas, engage in intellectual and social challenges. Share and drink from the collective pool of energies and emotions. Being starved of this contact and relegated to Dr. Phil and Regis and Kelly, again, is just too much.

One Sunday morning, I'm feeling very ill. I sit staring at a banana. It is actually the easiest possible thing for me to digest, no matter what's happening with my body. I know that when I don't eat, I get weaker, dizzier. I know that, when I do, eating causes massive amounts of pain. I coax myself into very slowly eating half of it. I pick up the *Nsew York Times Magazine* from the kitchen table and start reading. Everything is horrifically depressing. I decide that it's not just me that's diseased; it's the entire world.

I sit in Susie's chair in my bedroom, too sad to even cry. The world is just so bleak and hopeless I want to escape. There's something about emotional depression brought on by physical pain that's worse than any kind of angst I've ever had. The interminability of it is unbearable. It hurts to move; it hurts to eat. The landscape outside the window is cold and grey; I can't even sit outside because it's minus twenty. My bank account is overdrawn; I'm too sick to work. The relief I used to find in studying and in academic engagement is now gone too. If this is life, I don't want it. It is actually hard to imagine a scenario more alienating than having my bodily control disappear. The truth is that no matter how fastidiously

I build padded walls of people around me, illness and disease is a process that is done alone—entirely by oneself. The isolation is at times unreal. January 2003 is the most painful and lonely month of my life. I know things have become really desperate when, watching TV, I feel a sense of extreme wonder and envy at the possibilities life poses for other people. I'm convinced that just walking around in public and making life decisions that involve getting out of bed are options that may never be available to me again. I get an email from a friend visiting another friend in Japan. Smiling pictures. Such possibilities seem unbearably distant.

I remember at some point during this period seeing an interview with Kathie Lee Gifford in which she complains about the paparazzi following her around. She looks into the camera and says emphatically, "Nothing's worse; there's just *nothing* worse than this."

As I spend each day in the fetal position, I think she may be mistaken. I painfully try to retain the enemas that are promising to be my cure. Even after I give up on holding the enema in for the day, I'm afraid to move in case even the slightest shift provokes the spasm and pain that leaves me screaming on the toilet again as blood, mucus, and diarrhea evacuate from my inflamed colon.

I do this for a month. Not a day or two, not a few hours. An entire month. There are brief moments of reprieve, but they are forced and fleeting. I am better. *My colon is pink and healthy. This is a flu; it's going to go away.* By the end of the month I am sitting in my doctor's office, and she says, "Julie, we're going to have to do another scope. We have to find out what's going on."

"No," I say. "I can't, I can't, no. I don't feel well, I just feel so, so sick."

And she says, "I know, Julie, but we have to see what's going on."

She assures me that it will just be a "flex sig," short for flexible sigmoidoscopy, meaning that they won't try and push the camera through my entire colon, just through the end part, the sigmoid colon.

It's Tuesday, and she squeezes me into her schedule for Thursday. First, before any of her other patients. I have to be at the hospital at 6:30 a.m. I don't sleep for two days.

Thursday morning, I lie in bed, sure that if I move I'll throw up. I take some Gravol, which combined with the fact that I haven't slept, makes me very, very drowsy. It's a typical Toronto January morning. Freezing and dry. Each intake of breath makes me gag.

My rectum feels really inflamed, and every time I move, I feel a heavy weight in my tense, spasming abdomen. As soon as the nurse walks me into the room with the gurney and instructs me to put on the hospital gown, I burst into tears. Exhausted, weak with the nausea of my colitis and steroid withdrawal, I just can't face this moment. My rectum is so swollen it hurts to walk and I can't face a scope.

"What's the matter?" the nurse asks, shocked.

"I think I'm going to throw up," I answer. It's not true. An honest answer would be more like *I'm so scared. Please, please, please, please don't make me do this!*

"Okay," she says. "Here's a basin."

I lie there in the hospital gown, clutching the basin. So frustrated, angry, horrifically vulnerable, and just feeling so profoundly ill.

Dr. Lane comes in with a big smile that I suppose is intended to be comforting but I take to be taunting.

"Hi, Julie," she says.

The nurse wheels me into the scope room. They give me the pain medication that I know won't work, and well, you know the rest. The difference in this case is that Dr. Lane suddenly decides that her diagnosis has been wrong all along.

She points to the screen. "Look at the patchiness there. Yes, that's definitely patchy. I think it's Crohn's disease."

It seems to me that pumping medication directly into my diseased colon, twice a day for many months, could likely lead to a "patchy" appearance. If certain sections of my colon were healed by the contact with the liquid anti-inflammatory, this patchiness would not necessarily mean I have Crohn's. As I'm lying there, I tell Dr. Lane my theory.

Later, in the recovery room she gives me a prescription to start the steroids again because the enemas are clearly not "holding" me. This time I agree to start the immune-modulator drugs like a good, compliant patient. The steroids will "hold" me until the immune drug has the few months it needs to teach all the little killer cells that my colon is not, in fact, a foreign invader but a friendly settler. It certainly doesn't feel that way to me.

People have this strange assumption that flare-ups of a chronic disease become easier to deal with as time goes by. That when you're sick *again*, this somehow is more tolerable than the first twenty times. As if it is a skill set that simply needs to be developed and applied. Perhaps it's the only way they can continue their lives without processing the depth and breadth of my pain, which is valid. I'm not exactly soliciting pity parties at the time (this comes later). But this idea is simply a constructed delusion, created for their peace of mind, not mine.

Really, chronic illness leaves me weaker every time. Damaged. Less able to cope with the same thing, that is usually an increasingly worse thing, every time it attacks me. In healthy moments, I am stronger, tougher, more powerful than ever before. But when sickness defeats my will and slams me into depths that mock what I once thought was rock bottom, there is no darker place. Nowhere where my vision of the exit is more obscured.

7. Into Battle... *Again*

So now we're back again, to that moment that's punctuated by the staccato *Snap!* of yet another emergency ward doctor's glove. This time, this doctor calls the nurse back in to my curtained booth so he can do a rectal exam.

"I had a flex sig last week." I say. "We know my diagnosis. Do you really have to do this?"

"Yes, I have to do it," he insists. "If I call the GI guys in here and they say, 'You didn't even do a rectal exam?' there'll be trouble. This is procedure."

So I roll over. When his finger emerges from my rectum, he looks at his gloved hand with disappointment. "Hmmm, there's not very much blood."

I'm not quite sure how to respond. I have told him that I'm having twenty bowel movements a day, despite being on sixty milligrams of oral steroids. I have told him that I'm bleeding, in intense amounts of pain, weak, dizzy. I have told him that my specialist instructed me to come in and get my medication intravenously. But now I'm not producing enough visible disease in the last two inches of my rectum to warrant his concern.

He agrees to get the specialist in internal medicine to come in. The medication specialist comes in and orders my meds and starts me on the IV steroids.

Dr. Elliot, the internal medicine doctor, bustles in late in the evening.

He immediately starts firing off questions with machine-gun speed. I answer as well as I can through my malnourished, weak haze. He leaves; I go to sleep.

I wake up in the morning to the nurse asking me to come to the station because my doctor is on the phone. I know that Dr. Lane is on her way to Cuba for a well-deserved vacation, so I'm surprised. They wheel me over and I pick up the phone.

"Hi, Julie, I'm at the airport."

I can hear the crackle of her cellphone.

"I just wanted to let you know that I've arranged a specialist for your care while I'm gone; she'll be coming to see you this morning. She knows your case history and I've also told her that, if they need to scope you, you'll need extra meds. I won't be back for a week and a half, but hopefully you'll be out by then."

I thank her, and we hang up.

I return to my stretcher to a nurse bringing me my medication in a little Dixie cup with a glass of water. I quietly and calmly inform her that she's made a mistake.

"I'm not supposed to be getting my steroids orally. It's supposed to be on the IV."

"No," she says matter-of-factly. "Dr. Elliot changed the order last night. He wants you to take your medication orally."

The rage wells up through my chest and spills out of my mouth.

"Fine. I'll take them. And when I vomit them up you can call Dr. Elliot and tell him!"

It's not an oversight. It's spite. Dr. Elliot has decided that I am someone who is wasting his time and needs to be taught a lesson. *Because I so clearly want to be here.* You're not even supposed to take steroids on an empty stomach. He didn't order me any food. I'm not even on clear liquids. And it is basic medical knowledge that oral meds don't work when you're too sick to absorb nutrients. *The little chemicals in the drugs need to attach to the little nutrients from your food to be carried into your bloodstream, doctor. Did you miss the first day of med school?*

Elliot is on a power trip. When I am feeling stronger later in this hospitalization, I secure a private moment with my chart and read his analysis. It is peppered with "patient thinks" and "patient claims"; the deep sighs and eye rolls have practically become text. He makes a generous offer to "keep her for two days." Try two weeks.

I can understand that the ER should be kept for "emergencies." But considering, as Dr. Lane told me during my last hospitalization, that this is the only way in, you'd think a doctor might be more conscious of the fact that serious illness can encompass more than profuse visible blood, neck injuries, and heart attacks. It seems that the criteria is "Will she die tonight if I don't admit her?" And I doubt I would have. But the toll on my body and psyche is mounting quickly.

When the specialist that Dr. Lane arranged to see me comes in, I tell her about Elliot changing the order. She tries, quite unsuccessfully, to disguise her fury and immediately rushes out to change the order back to IV. I still have no idea why, but even though Dr. Lane sent her to take care of me, once she leaves my booth, I never see her again. She's written orders to admit me, so now it's just back to the waiting game for a bed in a room to become free.

While I'm still waiting on my stretcher in emerg, the space shuttle *Columbia* crashes. Or, more specifically, disintegrates, forty miles above the earth. It's not that I actually think that there are cosmic powers spinning all about just to determine world events based on clever ironies in my life. I just think that it's generally remarkable how if this were a fictional account, all of these parallel events would seem to be witty devices, to make some kind of dramatic point. But my life has turned into its own novel. I just have to recount the events as I see them unfold.

I am carted into Room 511. In a massive hospital with hundreds of rooms. The bed that they have brought me in from the emergency ward gets positioned in the Bed 1 spot. February 2. Two months after my first admission into this hospital, exact same spot. In the film *Groundhog Day*, Bill Murray repeats the same day, February 2, over and over until he gets it right. This is clearly my Groundhog Day. The doctors will have to try to get it right this time.

8. Conspiracy

"Are you girls conspiring?"

Dr. 40-Scopes looks honestly worried as he comes back into the room with Ali and me after rounds. Without a doubt, we are his most "challenging" patients this particular afternoon. Ali has a series of autoimmune conditions, many of which have symptoms I can't even imagine. This particular flare-up includes constant vomiting caused by toxicity in her organs. The only care is palliative until the attack passes. But it is not our diagnoses that are the problem for Dr. 40-Scopes. The real source of conflict is that neither of us can bother with the show of ingratiating ourselves to the Wise Doctor.

He greeted me earlier that day with an enthused "Hey, Sport!" as he bounced himself down on my bed, clapping the top of my thigh with his hand. I winced at the impact of his bounce on my inflamed nether regions. He didn't notice. It didn't really matter what anyone said to him, he was like a happy robot, the evil boyfriend Joyce Summers brings home in the *Buffy* episode "Ted," all salesman platitudes and clichés. So when he walks back into the room to find Ali and me talking quietly and laughing behind our curtains, it is with distrustful gravity that he asks, "Are you girls conspiring?"

"Yes," I answer, straight-faced. "Always."

He quickly gives Ali something that he forgot, an order of some sort or another, and shuffles out quickly without making any further eye contact.

A different specialist once told Ali that she was an "instructive patient." He was giving what he thought was a kindly warning that her reputation preceded her, and that this was not a way that she would want to be known. She calmly responded that she's been dealing with her disease process for over twenty years, so if she feels a clinician requires "instruction," then she feels compelled to give it.

Through this hospitalization, we become fast friends. Her husband, Carl, and Blair hit it off too. Sometimes when the four of us hang out in the room, watching TV or just chatting, Ali and I can pretend for a few brief moments that we are in some kind of civilized environment, a café, a living room, anywhere that isn't the starched sheets and stale air.

Our room is so hot that when the fan blows, it seems to be blowing hot air. My only reprieve is to close my eyes, adorn my lips with citrus balm, and pretend that I am in Hawaii. It's very effective. When I can imagine things vividly, being sure to include the most minute details, it really is as good as being there. The beach sand is white; my toes sink into its warmth. The ocean laps with force, daring and welcoming at once. The air smells like salt and, well, citrus lip balm. The curtains around my bed are bright orange and yellow, and they move peacefully with the breeze. Sometimes it seems that there is no real difference between thinking and doing, if you think something through long enough.

One day, while I am doing this, Uncle Tony calls. He sympathizes about how overheated hospitals always are. I explain my Hawaii method, and he's pleased.

"It's great to have an imagination."

But no amount of imagining reduces my anxiety about the fact that I'm going to endure yet another scope. Uncle Tony suffered his share of invasions in his last hospitalization.

"They've got to be sick," he says. "Those doctors just love doing their scopes."

He promises to visit me, if not in the hospital, then when I get home.

A week passes, and I'm not getting any better. If anything, I'm feeling worse. The excess cortisol racing through my veins from the steroids expands my face practically beyond recognition. My body is shrinking and shrinking; I'm melting like the Wicked Witch of the West. I've lost twenty pounds since Dr. Lane weighed me in her office.

I've always felt anxious about friends losing weight. I feel a sense of solidarity with similar female body types, and on some level, the skinnier they get, the further they get from my club, and into the VIP lounge of thin women. It terrifies me too, though, as if the overall movement of losing substance from their bodies will ultimately conclude with their complete disappearance. Invisible women, eaten from the inside out, wasting flesh, potential.

I flippantly say to the nurse, who looks horrified when she weighs me, "Well, every cloud has a silver lining."

She looks at me intently and scolds, "This is *not* the way to lose weight."

I am bounced back and forth between Dr. 40-Scopes and Dr. Bird as they come on and off shift. Neither of them can explain why I'm feeling so sick, except to ask accusingly why I'm not eating when they see my food trays untouched.

"Because I feel really, really nauseated. Isn't there anything I can have for this pain?"

Dr. 40-Scopes tells me again in a singsong voice that any painkillers other than Tylenol are bad for my GI tract. He orders Ensure to come with my meals and lectures me about taking my vitamins.

Dr. Bird comes by with the cover of a book he wants me to read. I've already read it. He looks surprised. When I ask him why I'm feeling so much worse, he deftly changes the subject.

"Well, if someone had started the immune drug two months ago, she would be in remission right now."

How can I possibly respond to such a bizarre, hypothetical accusation?

I'm already feeling guilty enough about the trouble my rebel colon is causing.

When Dr. Singer, the surgeon, drops in to see me, he is his usual friendly self. I tell him that I just keep feeling sicker, every day. Woozy, toxic.

He looks up at my IV bag that contains the liquid steroids.

"That's an awful lot of steroids for an awfully small woman. The dose is too high." He says this very quietly.

"Well, can't you get them to lower the dose?" I ask desperately.

"I don't want to step on anyone's toes. It's not my decision."

So I find myself wading through the minefield that is doctor egos. My mental power is fading. When Maia is visiting one day, she refers to a conversation we had the week before. I have no idea what she's talking about. No amount of prodding gives me the vaguest recollection of the details.

Ali and I always have tons of visitors. One day she comments how nice it is that all my friends and family are constantly phoning and coming in. But this isn't what I want attention for. They should be coming to hear me give a talk or to do something smart. Not visiting me during my fourth hospitalization in less than a year. I feel like the corpse in a casket at an Italian funeral, with streams of aunts and uncles coming to pay their respects. I lie in embarrassing discomfort, seeing my reflection in their concerned and sometimes frightened eyes.

It's during this hospitalization that my mum and I start discussing the possible causes of autoimmune responses. She developed an antibody in her blood while she was pregnant with me called anti-Lewis A. There are several theories on the origins of autoimmune responses in people. One is that there is a problem in the perinatal stage of fetal development. T-cells that are supposed to distinguish between what the immune system needs to fight and what it doesn't are not properly developed.

The bodily changes that happen to a woman during pregnancy can also lead to autoimmune conditions. After I was born, my mum had a flare-up of multiple sclerosis (MS). The doctors explained that there had been damage to the myelin sheath but that is was difficult to determine the cause of the MS and that it could only be proven by an autopsy of the brain. He was also concerned that another pregnancy could precipitate a more severe attack. Since then, she has had some generalized symptoms such as fatigue, weakness, memory problems, and occasional difficulties in swallowing. Because she continued to have minor relapses, her condition was ultimately diagnosed as a relapsing-remitting course of mild MS. Then, in her early fifties, she developed ulcerative colitis, another autoimmune disease. So what happened in the dark days of 1979? Something in my formation forever changed my mother's body, her immune system turning against her. And twenty-four years later, here I lie. Antibodies, antigens, autoimmunity.

Ali, who has a degree in biochemistry and is a diagnostic technician by trade, contributes heavily to these conversations. One day, an intern comes into our room to take my history for his chart. He's very nice, so I don't mind that it's about the thirty-seventh time I've given these exact details. I decide to talk to him about our somewhat undeveloped theories. He is very interested and tells about a study going on at the University of Alberta that's testing the genetic link between Crohn's disease and MS. He also mentions that immune-medications that work for Crohn's are now being tested on MS patients and encourages me to keep researching these connections.

Besides all of this heavy intellectual speculation, there's also much indulgence in bad television. The hospital doesn't get the Space Channel, so I can't hide in the comfort of *Buffy* repeats. Ali and I religiously follow *American Idol* auditions and the gripping plot twists of the first-ever *Joe Millionaire*. Daytime talk shows obsess over the details of each exciting reality TV show minute, making us feel almost as if we are engaged in something important—a pleasant shift from the pain, boredom, and helplessness that characterizes the rest of our days.

9. Now I Know How Joan of Arc Felt

Dr. Lane finally returns from Cuba. When she walks into my room, I am cramped up into the fetal position on my bed. I feel like someone just handed me an oxygen mask. I inhale deeply and tell her that I feel like I have eaten the contents of a giant car battery. I have no restraint about telling her exactly what Dr. Singer said.

She reduces the steroids.

"And by the way," she says, "you were right."

I look up, surprised, with no clue what she's referring to.

"The patchiness I saw on your scope was caused by the enemas. You don't have Crohn's disease."

It's so complicated. Some cases are really easy to diagnose because they clearly fit the symptoms of either Crohn's *or* ulcerative colitis. Mine mostly appears to be ulcerative colitis, meaning bowel ulcerations in the mucosal lining of my colon and nowhere else, but sometimes, like when it appeared patchy in the scope, it looks like Crohn's. Crohn's disease is the more serious of the two diagnoses because it can affect the entire digestive tract and there's no known cure.

Dr. Lane just spent a week and a half in Cuba. My scope was one week before that. The fact that she even remembered what I said is shocking enough. The fact that she has no qualms about admitting that I said it floors me, especially after dealing with the Old Boys' Specialist Club while she was gone. How did she escape medical training—who let her slip through the cracks? I take her admission as irrefutable evidence of her brilliance. She's smart enough not to feel threatened by the theories of a patient.

I know I'm definitely feeling better the night I go into the hallway with my IV poles demanding that someone come and give Ali her Gravol.

I am just so angry.

Ali has tubes for draining, surgically inserted through her nose, and feeding and medication through a series of tubes in her neck. A morphine pump allows her to self-administer painkillers. The problem is that the morphine makes her nauseated and she's not allowed to self-administer Gravol.

It's so basic. She needs the Gravol every four hours, so she can push the morphine button without another vomiting attack. She needs to take the morphine regularly, before the onset of more pain. Once the pain starts, the morphine doesn't work.

She's in pain. Horrible, unceasing pain.

I march into the hallway, carting my IV poles to the nurse's station. The nurse preparing the meds is talking and laughing. She looks at me impatiently and says she'll be there in fifteen minutes. But she's already half an hour late.

I've witnessed repeatedly that, because Ali has such specific needs, some nurses have labelled her a "whiner" and sought to exert their authority wherever possible. While Ali is absolutely not a whiner, and while this is not the opinion of most of the nurses, it only takes one on the night shift to cause a night of excruciating pain for Ali.

So I stand there. Glaring at her.

"She needs it *now*." I know that the nurse knows exactly what the situation is, but I explain it again. "She's in a massive amount of pain. She needs her Gravol before she can administer the morphine; otherwise, she'll be vomiting all night. It's already half an hour late."

I stand there, poles in hand, until she follows me back to the room with the Gravol. I need an extra sedative to sleep that night. The next day, I see in the chart how she's explained my nighttime behaviour. "Patient was awoken because roommate was disturbing her and would not stop screaming. She could not get back to sleep."

The next day, Ali tells her husband, Carl, of our escapades. He is furious with the nurse.

"Nobody would get away with this in a business. If I did this at work, I'd get fired."

I can only imagine the profound rage he's experiencing, seeing his partner in wild amounts of pain and knowing that there's a simple solution. Also knowing that he's explained this simple solution—repeatedly—and that the people who are granted the power to administer it are constantly acting as if it's no big deal. It is easy to become desperate, looking for solutions. Carl's conclusion is that we need privatized health care, run like a business.

And it makes perfect sense. I consider his words in silence for about four or five seconds until scenes from Michael Moore's television show, *The Awful Truth,* flood into my mind. Where private health care means that for-profit corporations decide what treatment is necessary and who is eligible for it. The horror stories are endless. And as it happens, I have a story of my own.

I attended an Ontario Progressive Conservative Party convention in 2000, when Mike Harris was still premier. I happened to be in the building where they were meeting, and I was wearing a suit jacket with a name tag that had someone else's name on it. Right. So without getting into the how's and why's—which are probably best left out of print—I saw Michael Walker, from the right-wing think tank the Fraser Institute, speak. He said,

"We're driving better cars than we've ever driven, living in bigger houses than we've ever lived in. So why should we have to line up with everyone else for health care?"

He congratulated Harris for all his cuts to health care (which I believe were made in the name of "efficiency") and for paving the way to privatization. He went on to encourage the Conservatives to take the next step—sell all these services to private industry so that he, his rich friends, and their families would never have to wait for health care again. Those with the fattest wallets would always be first in the queue. The media were blacked out from this event. The disadvantage of this was that I couldn't enact my plan because without the media to cover it, it would've been me versus the several hundred cops guarding the doors from the outside protests. Not the kind of odds I like. The advantage was that I heard what they discuss when no one is listening. I learned that while governments talk about "efficiency" in public, and about value for taxpayers' money, they are openly speaking in private about shutting out anyone who doesn't have the income to pay for their health.

Even as I'm recounting my tale, Blair is repairing the suction machine on the wall next to Ali's bed. The nurses have repeatedly phoned for someone to fix it, yet no one has come. So Blair is happily solidifying his reputation as MacGyver, the resourceful agent from the old TV show.

Carl still doesn't agree. He tells me how they've travelled to other countries and paid for experimental treatments for Ali's rare disease, and the way they were treated was a million times better.

But, of course, small, very well-funded facilities have better conditions. The problem is that *everything* should be that well resourced, not just places that most people would have to re-mortgage their homes to pay for. Publicly, politicians love to blame the victim whenever they make cuts to social services. "It's all these people going into the ER, blocking it up when they don't really have anything wrong with them." I remember a lot of bizarre talk in the 1990s about all the irresponsible people going to hospitals when they just need a Band-Aid. But behind closed doors, it's clear that they are simply interested in reducing taxes for the upper echelons of society so they can pay out of pocket for services that the rest of us will never be able to access. Then billions of dollars are taken out of health care budgets across the country, wait times increase, emergency wards overflow, and we're desperate for corporate saviours to come and rescue us. It's a consciously manufactured crisis.

I challenge anyone who argues that these policies are "good for the economy" to spend five minutes in my restraints closet in BC or to stand next to Blair as I am ignored, abruptly ravaged, and then discharged. The problem with our health care system is that it's not public enough. The hospitals are running on skeleton staffs. Creeping privatization, with assaults on working conditions and cuts to essential services, is giving us a glimpse of what privatized care would look like for the vast majority of people who couldn't pay for the Cadillac service. Then when we complain, privatization is offered as the only feasible solution. The scary thing is that it can quite easily appear to be true. Atomized inside the moments of personal interactions, it's hard to see the bigger picture.

10. A United Underworld of Anti-Julieness

They're pushing me down the hall for my final scope with Dr. Lane. In the hallway, I pick up my chart and start reading it. Dr. Bird's notes when I was first admitted read "Some abdominal discomfort, cushnoid face, obese abdomen."

My mum, looking at my body that has been slowly shrivelling up for the past two months, insists that it must be a typo.

"They speak into little tape recorders, and then someone transcribes it. He couldn't have said that. They must have heard it wrong."

"Mum, seriously, what rhymes with obese that could describe an abdomen?"

I personally think the good Dr. Bird can't tell the difference between my widely situated hips and excessive body fat. As I continue reading the chart, I see that he described my presentation in the ER as "some abdominal discomfort." I want a sledgehammer and five minutes to show him how *some* abdominal *discomfort* feels.

I put the chart down and Dr. 40-Scopes walks by, flanked on all sides by adoring interns. He shouts over his shoulder, "Hey there, do you like how puffy your face is?"

I glare at him. "Yeah, I love it."

He laughs appreciatively, as if we are having some kind of in-joke.

It's apparently funny to him that the dose of steroids he put me on, which left me feeling toxic for two weeks, is now tricking my body into retaining so much water that I have developed what those in the medical field sensitively describe as "moon face." I am not only a "sport," but my facial features have been stretched, obscured. The person I present to the world is being forcibly changed by medication.

And despite my staunch belief that more resources and better working conditions could heal many interpersonal conflicts between hospital staff and patients, I still think the problem of health care professionals' manners (or lack thereof) cannot be resolved with money alone. Not by privatizing, not by more public spending. It's not even about more training; it's about *different* training. Bucking against the historical flow of teaching doctors that they're the experts, called to manage patients' unruly diseases and bodies. It's about taking this patronizing attitude out of nursing schools too. A whole new set of skills needs to be taught—collaboration, respect for people's insights about our bodily experiences, nurturing kindness as daily practice. I believe this atmosphere would better serve health care professionals in their own learning and work environments. Bodies should never bear the brunt of anyone's competitive attitude.

Dr. Lane discharges me, with a high dose of steroids. The immune-modulator that I've been taking for the past month will not start working for another eight weeks. At this point, I'll be allowed to gradually start reducing my steroid dose. The immune drug makes me extremely nauseated. The only way I can tolerate it is with Gravol. Dr. Lane is insistent that the dose needs to be split: half with breakfast, half with dinner. The problem is that Gravol puts me to sleep.

So my life looks like this: wake up. Put in Salofalk suppository. Take Losec to control the acid reflux caused by the Prednisone. Have breakfast. Take Gravol to control the nausea caused by the Imuran. Take Imuran. Take calcium and vitamin D to control the bone loss caused by the Prednisone. Go back to sleep because the Gravol makes me drowsy. Have lunch. Take the Prednisone. Have dinner. Take iron for the anemia caused by the colitis. Have snack. Take Gravol and Imuran. Insert my second Salofalk suppository. Go to bed.

I am discovering that pharmaceutical manufacturers have their marketing strategies unashamedly revealed in the quality of their pills. So I develop new expertise: when faced with a generic pill, like Prednisone, for example, do not be fooled by the size of the pill. Prednisone is tiny. This is just as well, as it is made in five-milligram doses, which means taking twelve pills at this point in time for me. But despite their smallness, they are not easy to swallow. If attempting to swallow one, make sure your tongue is as dry as possible. This may require absorbing your saliva on a tissue. Put the pill(s) directly on your tongue and immediately swig ice-cold juice or some kind of sweet drink.

Pills that still have patent rights bring in the biggest revenues. As such, they are marketed so that they are more appealing to doctors and patients. They are packaged in attractive, convenient packs and coated to make them incredibly easy to swallow. They are accompanied with all kinds of safety information, labelling, and warnings. Products that are around long enough to be made by generic manufacturers come with no such extras. The pills themselves are not coated and the chemical process is in no way disguised in their horrific taste. If they contact any moisture, they instantly dissolve and become tacky, sticking to your tongue.

Generic pharmaceutical manufacturers have no need to market, for two reasons: the medication is already known to doctors and will be prescribed regardless of advertising, and there is not as much money to be made now that any company can produce it. The highest profits come from the cheapest method of pill production and the resulting unpleasantness for the patient.

At some point, I realize I need to address the pile of mail looming. Unpaid credit card bills and a letter from the company who insured my graduate students' health plan informing me that I exceeded my $2,000 drug maximum halfway through the year. The biggest expense that pushed me over the financial (as well as emotional) edge was to pay for the torturous enemas. It's pretty clear to me that I will easily accumulate the same costs again in the second half of the year. What is not clear is how I'm going to cover these costs.

Even more surprisingly, there are nasty letters from the naturopath, threatening to pass my account on to a collection agency and ruin my credit rating. And they're not just from some overzealous office administrator; they are signed in pen by her personally. The only reason I'm being billed after the fact is because *their* credit card machine broke down while I was trying pay. I immediately send a cheque with a pointed reply suggesting that, in future, when they're billing someone and that client is critically ill, it might be prudent to phone before sending letters—if just to create the appearance that they care more about health than monetary gain. I instruct them to close my account after her supplements made me sicker.

There are also repeated emails from the instructor of the distance education course I enrolled in. I decided while wallowing in illness a few months earlier that I wanted to teach college. So I applied for a distance education program at a university a few hours from home where I could train to do this. Now I'm going to fail if I don't submit my assignment right away. My mum was nice enough to phone the program for me while I was in hospital to explain, and they'd already agreed to put a hold on my registration until the fall. When I email back to explain, the instructor sheepishly apologizes for the mix-up.

I have a follow-up appointment with Dr. Lane, and she immediately understands the problem with my split dose of Imuran and subsequent inability to do anything. I bring a proposed medication schedule and she agrees. We move the entire dose to bedtime.

I buy another book about nutrition. This one has all kinds of information about soluble fibre. Apparently all of those white things (bread, potatoes, rice, etc.) are extremely useful for digestion in inflamed guts. They absorb acid and gently expand the colon to allow other things to pass through more comfortably. The "healthy eating" trend of eating coarse and raw fibre all the time doesn't apply to those of us with violent digestive ailments. Cutting out these "whites" wasn't just unpleasant psychologically, it wasn't even wise for my gut. Thank you, nasty naturopath. The most comforting thing I still carry with me from this book is not to feel pressured into dietary choices because of other people. The author strongly believes that we are best equipped to make gentle and nurturing decisions about our own bodies. This is also when I learn that you need all the little nutrients carrying the little drug chemicals through your bloodstream, and it renews my rage against Dr. Elliot, the doctor who refused to give me my meds on IV and sent oral meds without ordering food.

It's as if there was some twisted collusion happening between the ER doctor and the naturopath. A United Underworld of Anti-Julieness. First she denies me food. Then, when that doesn't work, Elliot launches in with attack plan B. I can picture their super-villain costumes. She's clad entirely in hemp, and he's wearing a sterile white military uniform and carrying a machine gun loaded with steroid pills. But they are ultimately outwitted by the forces of Good. In true comic book style, I am rescued, saved at the last possible second from the nefarious plots of my foes—until next time.

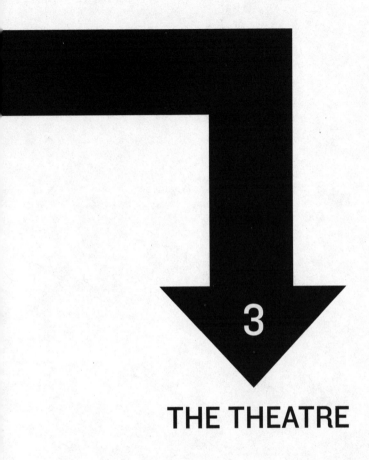

3

THE THEATRE

I. Casualty

And death shall be no more, comma, Death thou shalt die.
Nothing but a breath, a comma...not insuperable barriers,
not semicolons. With the original punctuation restored,
death is no longer something to act out on a stage, with
exclamation points. It's a comma, a pause.
— Margaret Edson expounding on poet John Donne's
"Death Be Not Proud" in her play *Wit*

The week I come home from the hospital it becomes clear that my little
dog, Susie, who I've had since I was ten, is very, very ill. She's become
so weak and skinny. She's throwing up, has diarrhea, and is extremely
confused. She's inexplicably staring at walls and looking into corners. I
can't handle another medical crisis. I pretend she's okay. I give her warm
baths and massages. I carry her around with me. I'm still not feeling very
healthy myself. I entice her to eat by feeding her whatever we're cooking
that she seems to like the smell of. She's refusing to even look at dog food.

I finally take her to the vet and they do some blood work. Her readings
are 18 percent of what they're supposed to be. I don't exactly understand
what this information means — no one's ever given me percentages like that

about myself—but obviously it's bad. They can't believe that she appears as well as she does, considering. I leave her at the vet's, to get rehydrated and to get medication for the pancreatitis that they've now diagnosed. They suspect that there's something more serious going on and want to do a four-hundred-dollar ultrasound to find out. I ask if whatever they might find is going to be treatable, and they say no. So I decide to just to treat the pancreatitis and see what happens.

I can't sleep while she's gone. I joke that she's getting her revenge for me leaving her to go to the hospital so often. When I phone to see how she is, the vet technician gets on the phone. Apparently, about an hour earlier, he took her outside and waited and waited while she refused to pee. As soon as he put her back in her cage, she stared defiantly at him and wet the blanket.

I laugh. "Wow, that's great!"

"*What?*" He's understandably confused.

"Well, she's got her spirit back; she must be getting better."

I understand why he might've been less than elated about Susie's resistance while dripping with her pee, but I can't help but be heartened that my little dog is still exhibiting her trademark attitude.

That's Thursday. Then one of the vets calls me late Friday night. She wants me to pick up Susie and take her to the emergency vet's where she'll be monitored overnight. Apparently her levels are dropping even lower and she's become critical. But I can't bear the thought that she might die alone there, wondering where I am and why we've all abandoned her.

So I'm sitting in the dark and empty waiting room. Desperately holding my dog as she licks the tears from my eyes and nose.

"She's coming home. I'm bringing her home."

"I really, really don't recommend that."

"I can't pick her up now and leave her somewhere else, she'll be so scared."

"Well, there are some things you have to watch for if you take her home. If she can't move or you notice fluid buildup in her joints, take her straight to the emergency clinic."

So against the vet's advice, I take her home.

She's so happy that whatever disease is ravaging her body is almost imperceptible. The anti-nauseants and anti-inflammatories are working, so she's really hungry but we don't want to aggravate the pancreatitis, so we don't feed her. I spend the evening researching Susie's illness and the night with her lying next to me in bed, sleeping while I massage her and watch her breathe.

The next morning, I take her back to the vet's to put her back on fluids and get her meds intravenously. In the afternoon, we have an appointment with our regular vet, Dr. Leela, who wasn't working the night before. She's glad that I took her home the night before; she feels it was the right thing for Susie's spirits. Then she looks at us gravely and tells us that despite all the interventions, Susie's blood counts have continued to drop.

"But can't the anemia be caused by the pancreatitis?" I ask desperately. "Maybe that's all that's wrong with her...it might not be anything else."

I explain that she has just been really stressed out because I've been sick. She gives me the same look as Dr. Lane does when I'm explaining that, this time, it's really not a flare-up of my colitis. Serious, sad. She tells me that it's cancer. That she must've had it for a long time to be so sick. She was probably putting on a brave face because I wasn't well. They can give me palliative medications and we can take her home.

So we do.

I can't handle the idea of watching her slowly fade away. To wonder every time I wake up or come home if I'll find her dead. I decide that Monday morning we'll put her to sleep.

Dr. Leela phones Sunday morning. I tell her my decision. She tells me that I'm brave and doing the right thing for Susie. Susie is still peppy on all the drugs, but quite obviously ill, nonetheless. We feed her small amounts every two hours to minimize the stomach upset. She thinks this is how mealtimes should have always worked—frequent and served in bed. I have a live wake for her that evening, so people can say their goodbyes.

Early Monday morning, we drive to the vet's office. I bring her organic lamb jerky because I know that's how I would want to go, munching on my favourite food. Dr. Leela gives her the injection, and she falls asleep, looking regal in her plaid sweater.

And it occurs to me that this is how everyone should die. Happy, on their own terms. Before taking her last dose of painkillers and ending her pain forever, artist Frida Kahlo wrote in her diary, "I hope the exit is joyful, and I hope never to return." It seems that sometimes we treat domesticated animals more humanely than humans. As a society, we are more adept at containing their suffering than our own. And the immediate comparison is even more chilling. I get sick; I have to fight for treatment. My dog gets sick; whatever care she needs is instantly available. Another specious argument to privatize health care. Except that just for a few days the bills are in the thousands. Luckily, family and friends make contributions, so I don't end up needing to fulfill the payment plan I worked out with the vet. I would have been making sizable monthly payments for nine months, otherwise.

The day we put Susie to sleep, I get an urgent message on my cellphone from the naturopath. I expect it to be an apology for their insensitive letter, but instead she's asking me to call her right away because she's sure I couldn't have had an allergic reaction to anything she gave me. But I don't.

I write an obituary and make memorial cards to send to friends and family. For years to come, I have dreams that Susie somehow survived the injection, and I have to explain to everyone that she didn't actually die and the cards were a mistake.

Two days later, I have my first appointment with a psychiatrist. I used to fantasize about seeing one, imagining indulgently lying on a couch and picking through my every thought, impulse, and desire. But when the moment comes, I end up taking it as more of a challenge to convince him that I am superwoman, dealing so incredibly well that my psyche is impenetrable. It works. I tell him about all my plans; I am enthusiastic, optimistic. I'm not sure if I'm lying to him, or just giving him a version of the truth based on lies I've already told myself. I leave out the part about the months I spent wanting to die.

Thinking back to Vancouver, when the images of blood pouring from my slashed wrists used to frequently cross my mind, I wonder now if it was less a matter of actual desire for death and more a case of wanting the radical transformation that death symbolizes. I wanted *life* to be different. But, at the time, I buried these suicidal thoughts so deeply, dismissed them with such shame, there was no question that I could discuss them with this doctor.

"Well, you seem to be dealing with this very well" is his medical opinion. He asks me questions about school. "What are your papers about?"

At the time I think he's just bored sitting there listening to people in distress all day so he picks friendly arguments about industrialization, politics, globalization, and *I* get kind of bored because he doesn't seem to know much about any of it. Looking back, I wonder if the questioning about seemingly unrelated topics is some kind of assessment technique. If it is, apparently I pass. He writes me a referral to a natural sleep clinic to help me get off the sleeping pills my family doctor prescribed and tells me he doesn't think I need to see him again unless something else comes up.

A few days later, I'm sitting on the edge of my bed when Dr. Lane phones. While I was in hospital, she found me a disease specialist who she hoped would be able to provide her and me with some new insights into my illness. Now she's calling to talk about it. She opens really tentatively, gently saying, "I just wanted to let you know; I've asked Dr. Loveless to take over your case after you see him tomorrow."

"Oh, okay."

"It's just that you're such a problem case. I mean not you, you're not a problem..."

I laugh at her backpedal.

"I know, I know, it's my problem colon."

"Yes," she says with a little laugh. "You have a problem colon. I'm worried about you coming off of the steroids this time. He's a specialist in your disease and he's agreed to take your case. If the immune drug doesn't work, he'll know what to do."

I thank her and say that I understand.

"I just want the best for you," she says.

And we hang up.

I can't believe it. I've just gotten the "it's not you it's me speech" from my specialist. I'm pleased by the decency and respect she showed by phoning me at home but emotionally gutted that she'll be gone.

The next day is my appointment with the highly reputed inflammatory bowel disease expert Dr. Loveless.

I get dressed and changed and undressed and dressed again until I feel I'm in appropriate attire to see this prestigious specialist. I carefully do my makeup. Wash my face and redo it entirely. I imagine a big oak desk. I will sit poised and ask intelligent questions, taking copious notes in my book. I've taken the time to read several studies he's authored and looked into the clinical trials he's organizing. I want to like him. To effectively rebound from The Break Up.

I arrive. A nurse shows me into the examining room and asks me to change. So I'm sitting on a bed in a skimpy hospital gown when he walks in. He's nice enough, but there's no hope. Steroid-refractory colitis is the theme of the day. He vaguely discusses clinical trials, presuming I haven't already read every detail of everything he's doing. When I press for details, he's dismissive. Now we just have to wait and see if the immune drug works. And if it doesn't, it's the knife. Seeing as that was already the plan, I don't see why I had to trade in the warm and kind Dr. Lane for him and his expertise. I feel deflated.

My dose of steroids is still high enough at this time that I'm mostly functional. I'm working on my papers from the courses I took the previous term, and I get re-involved with some activist campaigns. A friend of Blair's is running a theatre, so he gives me no-stress, low-commitment ushering shifts to make some money. My sister, Joanne, gets into grad school at Columbia in New York. She's planning to leave the following September. She knows that Blair and I are vaguely discussing getting married.

"So why don't you do it in August?" she asks as the three of us are sitting in a restaurant eating one evening.

"Yeah," I say, "we could."

"It'd get you on my health plan," says Blair.

We all laugh because, despite being true and being a pretty good reason considering his awesome benefits, we recognize that we're not exactly being romantic. My sister and I take out a calendar and decide that Saturday, August 16, is the best day, but nothing is really decided.

On the weekend, Blair and I have been sleeping in. I roll over and say, "Seriously, let's get married this summer." We talk about some of the details, and we agree. Blair is not exactly the proposing type and I'm definitely not the type who wants to be proposed to, so this works well for us. In the coming days, I realize how very much I want this. A hope, a declaration that the future is bright—a focus on love and life.

One of the campaigns I'm involved in is in Montreal. I'm sitting with my friends Martine and Estelle and a few others, folding leaflets in a café one day when my cellphone rings. It's my mum, and she sounds terrible. She tells me that her brother, my Uncle Tony, has had a heart attack.

"But, he's okay, right? He's fine, right?" My brain is screaming. *No no no no no no! This is not happening!*

"Well, it was a major attack. He's in hospital. He's doing okay, but it was major. I just thought you would want to know."

I don't tell anyone because saying it out loud feels dangerous and, well, it might make it true. I cancel my plans to visit my friend Astrid, who's in med school in Ottawa, and go straight home.

The next day is Monday. I phone Uncle Tony in the hospital in the morning. The nurse answers the phone and gets him for me. He sounds tired and short of breath.

"Did I wake you?" I ask.

"No, no. I woke up in the morning, but then sometimes I just doze off again, you know."

"So, in other words, yes."

He laughs. "Well, yes, but it's okay."

I tell him about the campaign I was just working on. We talk about Quebec politics and second chances. He's ready to take his. No more working all the time. He has a new lease on life; he's going to start exercising, eating right. Things will be different.

"I'm getting on the treadmill and running five miles as soon as I get home!" he declares.

There's a dramatic pause as I wait for him to finish.

He laughs. "That was a joke! *Five miles?*"

"I didn't want to offend you in case you meant it." I'm laughing now too. I add, "Can I please come and visit you? I'll just lie and say I'm the youngest sister."

It's during the SARS outbreak in Toronto and only immediate family members are allowed to see patients.

"No, no, I don't want you coming in here, I'll see you when I get home. Come over for coffee."

"All right," I reluctantly concede.

"How's next Tuesday?" he asks.

"Yes, for sure, I'll see you then. Take care."

"You too. Bye."

And so we hang up.

Saturday morning he dies. Fifty-four years old. New lease on life. Another heart attack. Dead. Instead of chatting over coffee in his apartment the following Tuesday, I'm at the funeral home, packed out with his family and friends.

When people talk about death, the stereotype, the reaction of disbelief, always entails descriptions of how "alive" the person was. And this was certainly true of my uncle, bursting with conversation and intellectual challenges. It seems impossible that this would all be gone. That it could vanish in the instant between one heartbeat and the next.

My days are wide open at this point. Expanses of time that I don't always know how to fill. I write my paper for my political economy course. My professor is great. I changed my topic about every ten seconds, but he's patient and supportive. I missed all the deadlines for graduate applications while I was in hospital. I'm also concerned that September is looming fast, and if I have a flare-up, if the immune drug doesn't work, I really don't want the additional stress of arranging medical leaves. It's incredibly frustrating. I'm clearly capable of researching, writing papers, and participating in academic discussion, but the university bureaucracies function in such a way that intellectual ability and desire to learn simply aren't enough. There has to be a commitment to medical stability that I'm simply not in a position to make. The steroid withdrawal is not going as smoothly as my coursework. I'm sleeping a minimum of thirteen hours a day. I think this will pass. I swim, exercise, try to eat well when I'm not feeling too nauseated.

Websites for my disease advertise fundraising BBQs for pharmaceutical cures. They post the figures for the massive amounts of money that have been raised across the country in previous years. But all the money is going toward medical research. There are reports of medical progress in the quest to find the gene, but nothing is offered to practically improve my quality of life while I materially experience the devastation of my illness. My own poverty has me living at my parents' house at twenty-three, borrowing money from my mother to pay for my endless prescriptions.

I need financial support for Blair and me to get our own place so I can start piecing together a semblance of a life I would choose, instead of one where every financial decision is mediated by my failing health. Imagine if some of this fundraised money went into housing bursaries or academic scholarships. I also desperately want social support. I don't even care if it's related to my specific diagnosis. The social impact of frequent bouts of isolation, intermittent employment, uncertain income, and not being able to make plans are common to any chronic illness. While I have amazing friends and I often feel comfortable being ill in their presence, I fantasize about how lovely it would be if some of this fundraising money went into some kind of social place for people to hang out *while* we're sick. Somewhere that other people who I have things in common with can gather and we will all understand if someone just wants to lie on the couch or needs to be near the washroom.

2. Surprise!

I have to leave my part-time job early one morning because I get so dizzy I can't function. I'm ushering at the community theatre for a dance competition, dealing with wealthy parents and their bratty children speaking to me as if I'm their indentured servant. The fun part is that neither of the bosses actually cares what these people think, so we have some latitude in dealing with them. But, today, it's all just too much. I go home, take some Gravol, and go back to bed.

That afternoon, Maia and Blair insist that I go out with them. I'm still feeling really woozy, so I don't feel like leaving the house, but I'm also worrying that we'll run into someone from work and they'll think I'm not actually sick. In the end, they manage to talk me into it. It turns out that they're taking me to my surprise birthday party. I had absolutely no clue, and am uncharacteristically speechless as friends from high school and university and political friends pour out of different corners and rooms. It's the Saturday night two days before my birthday, so a lot of my friends are expecting a fake sort of "Oh, my God!" when I open the door. They think there's no way I'll be fooled.

But they couldn't be more wrong. As I walk into the house, I'm just so confused. People who don't even know each other are all together. Ali and Carl, standing in the middle, grinning. I haven't seen Ali since we got out of hospital and hardly recognize her without all of the tubes and equipment. It's, without a doubt, a surprise. And it's very nice, normal, sweet.

A definite improvement on the kind of surprises I'm now becoming accustomed to. Like completely losing bowel control in the middle of a sidewalk in Halifax. I've always wanted to see the East Coast, so in the heady days of March, when my steroid dose is still high enough to convince me I'm well, I applied to a conference in Halifax to give a paper. It was part of my big plan to distract myself. My paper was accepted along with funding for my expenses. Maia had always wanted to go to Halifax, so she decided to join me.

The day before my paper, we go to a restaurant downtown and walk back to the place we're staying. It's raining, and there are giant lawns between the sidewalk and the big, blank, grey buildings and people's homes we're walking past. I know I need a washroom, but I think if I just walk faster, it will be okay; I'll get back in time. But the cramping is too severe. It's a choice of either collapsing in pain or just surrendering and releasing it. So I do. I feel the gushing warmth fill my pants and unexpectedly feel a secure sense of relief wash over me. It's not evident to anyone else what has happened. The pain has subsided, and after taking a shower and washing my clothes, the incident is over. When I get out of the shower and tell Maia what happened, she's really happy for me. We laugh about the struggle for continence at all costs and how, sometimes, it's better just to let go.

The next day, I give my paper—well, notes for it anyway. My concentration is seriously deteriorating, and I've been incapable of actually getting the paper into proper academic format. It goes well, despite this. But I'm just so exhausted. I have several hours of relatively okay energy, but the rest of the day, if I'm not lying down, I feel like I'm going to throw up.

And what would a trip to another province be without visiting the ER? This time though, it's for Maia. One evening, we're sitting in the residence room and she starts breaking out in hives. Big, swollen, itchy hives, covering her entire body. Within minutes, her lips start to swell. We immediately get into the rental car and head to the hospital. Unspecified allergic reactions that entail oral inflammation get seen to very quickly. She's given an antihistamine and closely monitored for an hour and a half until the reaction has cleared completely. It mysteriously never happens again.

The next day begins with an argument.

"But I don't want a tattoo," I insist.

"Okay, but say you did, what would you get?"

"Nothing because I don't want one."

"Come on, you must have thought about it."

"Well, I suppose if I was going to get one, I would get a tiny ladybug on my right hip."

"And what if I was going to pay for it?"

So we get our tattoos. Maia gets the Chinese character for Earth on the inside of her forearm and I get my ladybug. I used to collect them in jars when I was little. Feeding them grass and then letting them go.

The tattoo artist is very thorough and meticulous in his questions, methods, and technique. When he disinfects the chair, gets fresh plastic gloves, and shows us the sterile seals on the needles and ink he's going to use, I tell him he's cleaner than some hospitals I've been in.

"Well, you hit the nail right on the head there," he says with an East Coast lilt. "My sister's a nurse and she couldn't believe it when the Department of Public Health rated us first and the hospital second."

He says this with an entirely straight face, and I can't help wondering if he means it.

We go to Pier 21 and see the actual doorway where passengers from ships in the 1950s arrived in Canada. Passengers like my mum and her family, arriving from Italy. My mum and Uncle Tony had both repeatedly told me the story of him throwing her doll over the side during the voyage. He was two and she was five. At the funeral, my mum's older brother spoke of how Tony had entertained the boat with his already magnetic personality and playfulness. I take pictures for my mum and get some souvenirs.

We take a rental car to Peggy's Cove. I become extremely nauseated and need to lie down. I sleep on the rocks as the waves come in and the whole way back in the back seat of the car. I spend the weeks following the trip in various states of sickness. The living room couch gradually becomes my permanent station. At some point in here, I have a dream. Uncle Tony is on what appears to be a TV screen, but it's really crackly, as if the reception is bad. He's green and his voice is breaking up. I keep trying to talk to him, but we can't understand each other at all. When I wake up, I tell my mum.

"I don't care if he's purple next time!" she says. "You stay there until you figure out what he's saying."

I make a pledge not to let her down in my next dream. My mother has always had a hilarious level of faith in what she believes to be my psychic abilities.

I phone the specialist, Dr. Loveless. His secretary, Laura, gives me an appointment for a couple of weeks later and says that, in the meantime, if I get worse, I need to go to emergency. My entire family takes turns sitting down at various points to tell me that I need to go to the hospital.

So mid-July, I am walking into the emerg at the downtown hospital where Dr. Loveless is based. There's a security guard at the door. She gives me a mask and disinfectant for my hands. She tells my mum that she can't come in because of the new SARS rules. This is my seventh emergency room visit in fourteen months, and now I am alone. By the time the triage nurse sees me, I'm in tears. I just feel so beaten.

"Why can't anyone come in with me?"

"I know, I know," she says, sympathetically handing me a tissue. "It's the rules."

They get me on a stretcher and on IV fluids almost immediately. The emergency doctor starts the "roll over" routine, but I refuse to comply.

"Dr. Loveless told me to come in. Everyone knows my diagnosis. The rectal exam is not necessary."

He looks at the nurse and shrugs. "Okay, we don't have to do it. I'll get the specialist in."

The first resident who sees me is super, really genuine and understanding. A few hours later, he comes back and we're talking when another resident comes bouncing in, looking like he's been sampling from the amphetamine cabinet. I'll call him Benny. He grins and flings his hand out to me, introducing himself. He ambushes me with question after question that I've already answered. I'm weak, tired, frustrated, and completely free of my fear of being branded a "difficult" patient.

I say nothing, impatiently glaring at the nice resident, who finally intervenes.

With an apologetic smile, he says, "He has to ask you himself to make his own assessment, it's just the way it works."

"Yup!" says Benny. "I can't believe anything this guy tells me!" He laughs loudly, slapping the nice resident on the shoulder.

I just roll my eyes. But, luckily, before we have to engage in direct combat, a specialist arrives. He's got an immediately comforting presence. He sits down and introduces himself. "Hi, I'm Dr. Gold."

He explains that he shares an office with Dr. Loveless and that he'll be treating me today. It's strange because in some ways I'm less sick than any other time I've come into the emerg. Yet in some ways, this is the scariest.

He's so gentle and respectful. We have the opposite argument of the one I've had in every other hospital emergency ward. He really wants me to stay in for the weekend, getting steroids and fluids on IV, but this time I really don't want to be admitted.

"I'm getting married in three weeks; I really don't want to stay here."

Both he and his resident smile warmly at this news.

"Congratulations," he says, with heart.

He gives me a new prescription for oral steroids and makes me promise that if it doesn't start working right away, I'll immediately return.

He looks at me with sad eyes. This hospital specializes in inflammatory bowel disease. Dr. Gold actually knows what I'm going through. I don't realize it until then, but sympathy scares me more than indifference. He understands that my past was wrenching. He knows that my future is the knife. It's kind of unbelievable that after spending so long trying to convince medical professionals that I'm actually ill, the ones who really upset me the most are the ones who unquestioningly accept the gravity of the situation. I find rage easier than fear.

In order to acknowledge how terrified I actually am, I have to accept my vulnerability, my lack of control over the situation. And this is not just humbling; it's more emotion than I even know how to process. So more often than not, I choose anger. There is certainly no shortage of incidents and people in my medical journey to fuel my rage. It gives me a sense that I'm still able to martial the ever-changing boundaries of my disease and body—that I still have the power to resist. Perhaps it seems ironic that, as a patient, I spend as much time dealing with feelings of anger as I do coping with issues of ill health. But I also believe this sense of righteousness is the tether that allowed me to keep my identity and not get entirely immersed and disappear in hospital-land. For this reason, sympathy is always a threat—and terror, its embodied accomplice.

It's the only somewhat positive experience in an emergency room that I've had so far. Ironically, it's the only time I get a follow-up questionnaire in the mail asking for feedback. The following week I get a phone call from the emerg doctor. The results of my stool sample have come back. I have an infection called *C. difficile*; he's going to phone a prescription of antibiotics into my pharmacy.

"So this might not have been a flare-up of my colitis?" I ask.

"Maybe not," he says.

I am massively relieved. I have another piece of evidence to carefully tuck into my denial file.

A few days later, I have my appointment with Dr. Loveless. In the days leading up to my appointment, I've been hanging out with my friends

Ethan and Astrid, who are med students. I constantly plague them with my cautionary tales of what happens to bad doctors. We discuss the mystery of autoimmunity and my frustration that medical science hasn't figured out why my immune system thinks the mucosal lining of my colon is a threat. All the research I can find being done is on genes or the search for ever-more obscure and strange pharmaceutical therapies. It seems to me if there is "a gene," I certainly have it, but it's unclear to me what knowing this will do to help my condition at twenty-four.

I want access to the research as it's being done. Be in their labs, looking at their data. Participating with a much more pressing motivation than just careerism. I ask my friends about the various research jobs they have had in labs and clinical trials and if they actually needed all the science they took in university or if they mostly learned as they went.

"Do you think my arts brain could hack it?"

"Oh, totally!" says Astrid.

Ethan nods emphatically, agreeing.

They are positive and encouraging.

So when I see Dr. Loveless, I ask if there's any research work I could be involved in. I know he's doing some big projects in the area, and I imagine that volunteers could be helpful. But I suppose there are science students bending over backwards submitting CVs to get these positions.

"What exactly would you do?"

He almost spits out the words, looking at me the way my immune system has been looking at my colon. Foreigner. Unrecognized, and unwanted.

"I could do anything you usually hire students to do. I mean, I don't just want to serve coffee."

He politely thanks me and says that he'll keep it mind before rushing out of the room. Just thinking about this moment still makes me blush many years later. I'm sure it made a great anecdote for him to tell his doctor friends—the epitome of the Uppity Instructive Patient.

When my course of antibiotics is finished, I'm still bleeding quite a bit, despite the fact that I'm still on the full dose of steroids. I phone Dr. Gold's office and leave a message asking for more antibiotics because I don't think the infection has cleared.

Dr. Gold phones me back himself, late in the evening, on my cellphone. He sounds terrible. No matter how angry doctors sometimes make me, they all strike me as being helplessly fragile. Hard shells, crumbling centres. I have a dramatic image of him sitting at his big oak desk and having a whiskey before he sat down to tell me.

"I think we need to consider the surgery sooner rather than later."

I am very calm on the phone. "Yes, I'll make the appointment with the surgeon. I understand."

As I hang up, I feel my chest dissolve into mush. The clay statue shattering with the first major blow.

This is when I enter what I call the Big Gestures period. Some people become very insular with such prospects. I decide two things: that if there was ever a time to do or say anything I had been afraid to do or say before, this is it. And that if there is ever a time that no one should be judgmental about such decisions, this is also it. Throwing large gestures in every direction, sometimes out of curiosity about how far I can push myself and other people, sometimes out of true desire. I also feel an overwhelming sense of defiance. If this is what my life looks like when I play by the rules, then the rules are clearly all wrong.

3. Wedding Feast (also, Fairies!)

The thing I remember most markedly from the month leading up to our wedding is how many people I don't know tell me I'm pretty, or even beautiful. And it's really odd. It's the first time in my life that I actually feel pretty. Even as medical professionals describe my face as "cushnoid," the rest of the world seems to see something else.

People keep asking me if I'm getting stressed with preparations, but not only am I having fun planning the biggest party of my life, I'm noticing how much easier it is to organize things that don't require fundraising, postering, meetings, and leafleting, and that are not only legal but socially sanctioned and praised. It's the easiest thing in the world to organize, and everything simply and easily falls into place.

I'm not someone who has ever acknowledged, even to myself, that I harboured wedding fantasies as a little girl. But when Joanne asks me in April, "Okay, but just for argument's sake, if you could have the wedding anywhere, where would it be?" immediately, the heritage house near my parents' house springs to mind. The property is beautiful, and the old white house regal and comfortable looking all at once.

"So call them," she says.

"Oh, they'll be too expensive."

"Well, you won't know unless you phone, and then at least you'll have some idea what venues charge."

So reluctantly, I do. It turns out that they're actually pretty reasonable. The house is owned and run by the township, which I didn't know at all, so they're not priced the way a private venue that beautiful would be. And, magically, this place that I've always wanted to get married in, has a cancellation for Saturday, August 16. The woman I speak to stresses how unusual this is because for a summer Saturday wedding people book two or three years in advance, not four months.

"The caterer is still holding the booking from the people who cancelled because she knew she'd fill it, so you'll have to make arrangements with her."

She gives me this woman's phone number and we arrange to meet. Her name's Michaela, and she's Sicilian. She's already met with another interested couple, but they haven't put down a deposit yet. So my parents, Blair, and I go to her premises and she serves us an amazing spread of wedding food that will suit all of our family and friends. My parents put down the deposit. When I initially told them we were getting married in August, they couldn't imagine a four-month turnaround. They kept insisting that we wait at least until the following spring. But I couldn't imagine spending an entire year talking about and planning a wedding.

And things keep magically falling into place. Like when I find the most amazing dress in the history of the universe. It's my friend Kara's birthday. We're meeting at her favourite restaurant, on Queen West, near Spadina. Another friend, Lia, and I meet on the subway to travel down together. Lia's sister got married the summer before, so she's still in the wedding-planning mindset.

"You don't have a dress yet?"

"Nah, haven't seen anything yet."

The dress issue isn't concerning me at all, but Lia is insistent.

"We're early. Let's just go into a few stores."

I reluctantly agree and follow Lia up the stairs into a Chinese dressmaker's on Spadina. They're closed, so I start to turn around. The owner comes out from her sewing room, across the hall from the display and store area.

"Come in, come in!"

She unlocks the accordion doors at the display area and waves us in.

"Do you know what kind of thing you're looking for?" Lia asks me.

"I'm not sure, maybe something silver."

"What about this?"

Lia pulls out a silver dress that, to me, looks like something a fairy princess would wear. Perfect.

"Oh that's a bridesmaid's dress," the dressmaker tells me.

"Do you care?" Lia asks me.

"No, not at all," I say.

She encourages me. "Well, try it on then."

I put it on, comfortably and easily. The dressmaker starts pinning up the bodice to fit me. To put the joy of this experience in context, the only other time I'd tried on wedding dresses, I went to a very fancy shop with another friend a month or so earlier. My arms didn't even fit into the sleeves of the tiny size four display versions.

I love this dress. A fitted silver boned bodice and a taffeta floor-length skirt covered in white mesh so the silver shines through.

I ask her to put it aside and promise to come back the next day.

The next day, I return with my mum and her younger sister, my Aunt Mary. When I put the dress on, they both exclaim, "Oh, Julie!" and Aunt Mary starts crying.

The dressmaker is oblivious to the excess of emotion spilling out around her.

As she continues pinning me into it and taking measurements, she demands, "How tall is your fiancé?"

"Um, six-two."

She looks up and down at my never-quite-made-it-to-five-four frame and declares, "You'll need at least three-and-half-inch heels."

Such an idea has never occurred to me. Other than jokes menacingly being told by tall friends that women my height aren't supposed to take the tall ones, I've never really considered our height difference.

A few days later, my sister takes me shopping in Yorkville. She discovers a pair of designer Italian leather silver sandals. The three-and-half-inch heel is a stylized kind of chunky that is comfortable as well as looking extremely feminine. As I affix the ankle strap, I'm in awe. My feet and ankles have never looked like this before. It's incredible how a pair of designer sandals can transform a pair of peasant grape-stomping feet. And they're on sale. Still, they're way beyond anything I could imagine spending on a pair of sandals.

My sister whips out her credit card.

"Joanne!" I try to restrain her. But she works out and she's stronger.

"This is my engagement gift," she insists.

And I can't *really* fight anyway; the shoes are beautiful.

Soon after, I get a phone call from Blair's mother. We small talk for a little while before she tentatively asks, "So what colour is your wedding ring?"

"It's yellow gold; it's my grandmother's, my dad's mother."

"Oh, well, I don't know if you're interested. I mentioned it to Blair, but I wasn't sure. My mother's engagement ring was yellow gold, and I still have it. Do you want it?"

"Yes!"

"Well, come over and see if you like it."

This conversation is emblematic about everything that's different between Blair's family and my family. When I speak to Blair later, I ask, "Did you know your mum offered you her mother's engagement ring to give to me?"

And he's shocked. "No, I had no idea."

"Do you remember her mentioning it?" I ask, now amused.

"Um, yeah, maybe..."

In my family, people wouldn't have hinted. In fact, they wouldn't have even just asked outright. They probably would have yelled it and somehow managed to pick a fight. And then it would become "the story about when I offered you my mother's ring," told repeatedly with new embellishments every time. So we go over to his parents' house that night, and his mother presents us with an incredibly beautiful diamond solitaire engagement ring from 1925. Blair slips it onto my finger with complete ease. It fits perfectly. We discover later that it matches my grandmother's ring exactly.

I walk around now with this gorgeous vintage ring on my fourth finger. I joke with friends that clearly some of my feminine social training took, despite all doubts to the contrary. For Blair's ring, we find a ring maker in the tiniest, most crooked shop I've ever been in. His name is Wolfgang. His wife's angel art is all over the walls. He takes out the tray of men's rings, and when I try to push one onto Blair's finger, he yelps and jumps back. I'm surprised.

"What's the matter?"

"It's where I had my surgery." He shows me the scar that I'd forgotten about—he was born with those fingers webbed.

The ring maker is intrigued by this new challenge.

"I've actually been working on different shaped rings," he tells us, "because when you think about it, no one really has round fingers."

He takes out some prototypes, and Blair, being a craftsperson himself, is totally intrigued. So they plot together about how to shape and design it, coming up with an incredibly cool plan that the ring maker creates Blair's wedding band from.

Maia and Joanne are my bridesmaids or, as I refer to them, my "best women." We go shopping for their dresses and they pick out ones they love enough to wear again. We go to a funky store where they both end up picking ball gowns: Joanne in forest green, Maia in lilac.

Now it's two days before the wedding, and the entire eastern seaboard is blacked out—a sticky hot night in Toronto with no air conditioning. Everyone but Blair and I seem panicked. We just trust that it's going to work out all right. We sleep outdoors, enjoying the view of galaxies normally obscured by city lights.

Bobbie flies in from Manchester the night before. She sits with us at the head table in a bright fuchsia dress. I love the spread of colours. Getting married is one of the least original things Blair and I will ever do, so I'm not very interested in making too much of a unique statement with our choices. The vows "richer, poorer, sickness and health, better or worse" all sound pretty good to me. They're classics for a reason. When people want us to kiss, they tap their glasses with cutlery. We like kissing; there's no need to tax our guests with arduous tasks. Our *Bonboniere* are candied almonds in white mesh flowers.

I had met the minister I want while doing peace organizing, and she immediately agreed to marry us. She ended up being on vacation, so she sends a man as a replacement who is much more conservative than she is. It works out in the end because if we're not getting married in a Catholic church, the family definitely prefer a more traditionally thinking man —and Blair and I are so giddy we barely notice. We've gone through the marriage ceremony and have made notes for him, some of which he takes, some of which he doesn't. At least at the end he takes my rewording and declares us "partners in life."

In the wedding video, while our witnesses, Joanne and Colin, are signing our wedding papers, we're standing in the back corner of the glass conservatory, pointing and giggling. In the entire video, with scenes of lots of people during lots of moments, there's a constant tinkling of laughter in the background. Blair and I dance our first dance to Tori Amos covering Led Zeppelin's "Thank You." It's a B-side from the first CD I ever borrowed from him when we were first friends. He made me swear to give it back and I still haven't.

The caterer checks in with me to give me updates every now and then. She says, "You're the most relaxed bride I've ever worked with."

"What's stressful about this?" I ask her. "It's the most fun thing ever!"

"The staff are having a really good time too," she tells me. "Your guests are great. And they're all talking about your dress in the kitchen. It's everyone's favourite of all the weddings we've done."

"Thanks!" I tell her. "You and your staff are amazing too."

I'm especially grateful that she's sent a beautiful Adonis of a young man to serve me all day. Like, literally, from right after the ceremony with a tray of appetizers to re-filling my champagne glass while I'm dancing with it in my hand.

We're surrounded by friends, families, and magical fairies in a beautiful old house that my friends have decorated with incredible love and skill. We feast and dance into the night. I can unequivocally say that this is the happiest day of my life.

4. Bionic Woman

"You're going to be bionic."

She looks at me with awe. We're sitting in a Vietnamese restaurant; my friend Estelle is having her lunch and I'm just drinking red wine. I laugh. This is why I called her. Her fascination with science makes her entirely impressed with every aspect of my pending surgery. Sympathy is the thing I can't handle. When you boil it down, it's essentially the sentiment "Christ, I'm glad I'm not her" — the polar opposite of the envy I presume we all actually crave.

Bionic Woman becomes my new title.

Two hours earlier this is the scene: the confident young resident strides in with a grin. He shakes my hand and briskly starts to take my medical history. All my practice at deference goes out the window as he addresses me with The Tone: The clever young man whose ego has been routinely stroked since birth. Now accomplished enough to be studying in a prestigious surgery program. Kind enough to bless me with five minutes of his time. Surely I should be trembling with gratitude. He starts firing off questions. He doesn't like how quickly I answer them. I'm sorry if my impatience with repeating every single excruciating detail of the last two years to someone who plainly doesn't care is becoming evident. It quickly becomes a medical duel. He's not liking that I know the Latin words, and he starts challenging me with more and more obscure and detailed questions. I rise to the fight…throwing his questions right back at him. The rhythm and tension of battle is rising.

"Do you know what the exact dose of Solu-Medrol you were on a year ago in hospital at St. Paul's?"

I start to say that after all my hospitalizations, it is difficult to remember such obscure details (which should be in my chart anyway), and he begins to smile triumphantly, opening his mouth to respond.

I cut back in, "I do know that the oral dose of steroids I was discharged on was thirty milligrams, I just can't remember the conversion rate from the liquid IV form offhand. What is it again?"

He looks flustered, "Well, it doesn't really matter. Have you been on any other medications this summer?"

"I started taking the birth control pill again because my symptoms are usually associated with my period. I asked Dr. Loveless if I should go back on the pill without allowing for breakthrough bleeding between pill packs to see if it helped me taper the steroids."

He laughs. Heartily and loudly. "Did Dr. Loveless think this was relevant?" he asks with a patronizing, disbelieving grin.

I have a flash vision of his textbook in my head. The lecture where the doctor smiles and tells them in a booming, authoritative voice that colitis patients develop all kinds of amusing theories about what causes their disease. And you know women, always making all kinds of unfounded claims about periods.

"Well, Dr. Loveless didn't know much about it. But considering that I read all the studies, including the ones where women only take courses of steroids during periods that cause flare-ups and not at any other time, he thought it was worth a try, if I thought not having periods would help. I already discussed it with my gynecologist. She thought it was relevant."

I think about women's ancient knowledge about our bodies and the scientific response: dismiss it out of hand, rediscover it, then take credit for it. Historically, midwives gave pregnant women castor oil to cause spasms in the colon to induce labour. Why wouldn't menstrual cramping be linked to inflammation of the colon and diarrhea?

I pause dramatically and lean toward him, "Why, do you not think it's relevant?"

"Oh, um, I don't know…" he mutters.

He backs out of the room. "I'll just go and get the surgeon now."

A few minutes later, they walk in together. I'm nervous about meeting another surgeon, but this quickly fades as she walks toward me and shakes my hand. "Hi, I'm Athena."

She pulls the chair toward me — the one that he sat in at a safe and objective distance. She opens my chart in her lap. "Wow, you've really had a hard time of it."

We talk about my master's program and my university. She knows so much about progressive politics that her young resident looks surprised. She laughs, waving her hand at him. "I dabble…" And then to me, "I have a friend who teaches women's studies."

She invites me into her office and shows me her medical books, describing in detail everything she is going to do. I trust her implicitly. I realize later that it is at least in part because she reminded me of Susie's final vet. It occurs to me that the surgeon may not receive this comparison as the huge praise it is.

"So we'll start the procedure laparoscopically, meaning, we can just cut little 'key holes' and insert cameras inside of you. We perform the surgery with long tools so you'll be left with only tiny scars. But after all the inflammation and the steroid medication, your colon might just be mush, in which case it could be dangerous to continue. In that case, we have to cut." At this point, she looks at me and cups her hands. "Because I would rather be able to hold it, and see exactly what we're doing if that's the case."

I feel safe for the first time in all the chaos and medical mayhem. She is going to hold my colon in her gently cupped hands.

It's the first time I've heard the word *ileostomy*. I feel a bit nauseated even typing the word. A piece of my small intestine, at the ileum, temporarily pulled out onto my abdomen. Emptying my bowel into a bag. Forced, surgically induced incontinence.

At this point I have another video art clip playing in my head, which I need you to picture. It starts with the word *cure*, and then an *s* and *d* come dancing in (okay, slightly *Sesame Street*-esque), and here's what happens:

Cure

cure

cures

s

Curse

CURSE

CURES

cured

CURSED

I think there's sort of a dramatic gong that lands on the word *CURSED*. Maybe Opera Guy can conduct the letters. Incidentally, Blair bought me a stuffed Opera Guy the first time we ever took a trip together, but this is beside the point.

The sort of unmitigated enthusiasm they all seem to have about the surgery being the cure to all my woes makes me nervous. It feels like the scene in the movie where the man tells his wife, "I'll be right back," just before he explodes into fleshy, gooey bits everywhere because there was a *bomb* in his car.

I want to believe her. We get back to the details of the surgery, when I might have the second one done. There are two main problems I run into with doctors: the first and most common is being patronized and not given enough information. The second is that, because I have fairly extensive knowledge about certain aspects of my disease, they assume that I have general knowledge of medical terms, and they go into Latin overload. As she starts to do this, I interrupt, trying to clarify what she is talking about.

The arrogant resident is thrilled with my demonstration of ignorance and tries to cut in to answer my questions. To her credit, the surgeon doesn't allow him to get a word in edgewise and patiently explains every detail without condescension.

I ask her about the development of other autoimmune diseases.

"My mum has ulcerative colitis. She also had multiple sclerosis. What's my risk of developing other autoimmune diseases? I'm also concerned about my joint inflammation. I understand that it's related to my colitis, but if my immune system is attacking my joints, why would that stop when you take out my colon? How is it any different from rheumatoid arthritis?"

"There's a very small percentage of the population that develops ulcerative colitis. There's a very small percentage that develops MS. The percentage that develops both is tiny. Your mum was just very unfortunate. Your joint inflammation is not the same thing as rheumatoid arthritis; when your colon is removed, it will go away. And, of course, we'll have to schedule you for a scope first."

I'm shocked. "Why?"

"I need to see for myself that it's not Crohn's disease."

"Can't you scope me just before the surgery, when I'm already unconscious?"

"No, we can't do that. We need to do it ahead of time to make sure you need the surgery. Don't worry. I'll make sure you have enough medication. I'll do it. We won't even start until you say it's okay and we'll stop anytime you say."

I am vaguely relieved. I do trust her and certainly want to know for sure that my diagnosis is correct before undergoing a major operation.

"You know," I say, "I'm more anxious about the scope than about the surgery. I've had some really, really bad scopes."

She and her resident exchange amused looks and surprised laughs.

I defend myself. "With the surgery, I'm not going to know what's going on. I don't care what you do when I don't know what you're doing. Scopes are traumatic, and the medication never ever works."

It is apparently unthinkable to them that the drastic, transformative intervention of *cutting me open* could be less frightening than a diagnostic test. But the invasion and violation of being scoped while awake and in pain is what keeps me awake in anxiety-filled nights.

"Don't worry, we'll check your chart. We'll make sure you get more medication than in your other scopes."

What can I do but agree? *You can only be cured if you agree to this procedure.* Is that consent?

She encourages me to schedule the surgery with her office administrator, and I leave to do so. I am relieved that this surgeon-goddess will be taking care of me. The office administrator is amazing, warm and genuine and open. We schedule the surgery for six weeks later. The surgeon wants to do it sooner, but there is simply no time in the schedule.

When I leave the building, I am on fire. Inflamed, in flames. Part of me thinks, *Of course this is the best thing; I'll get through this surgery, no problem.* Another part of me thinks, *Maybe this is it. Maybe I'll go under the anaesthetic and that's it. It's over. And what will I have missed?* It's a remarkably easy question to answer: Mexico City. Like any self-respecting young Canadian woman struggling through grad school with a chronic illness and a penchant for socialism and women's liberation, I want to see Frida Kahlo's house, go to the Trotsky museum, see the Rivera Murals, the studios. I want to feel Mexican sun warming my skin in a thriving, buzzing urban centre. Mad markets and bright colours. *¡Viva la Revolución!*

At first I push the idea from my mind. Then I ask Blair. "Would it really freak you out if I just up and went to Mexico by myself?"

"Yes." He glares at me.

To be fair to Blair, the steroids have already stopped working. My joints are becoming increasingly inflamed, and my digestion increasingly unpredictable. My energy is crap, and my mental state is questionable.

"Well, do you want to go to Mexico?"

"No." Blair once again answers curtly and directly.

I realize that I'm being unreasonable, but really, what's reasonable? My body is being decidedly unreasonable. I give it plenty of ultimatums, and it manages to deke them all out. Now, for the first time in a really long time, this will not be about me catering to an immune system gone wild. This is going to be about me.

So, without telling anyone, I go to the campus travel agency.

"Do you have any cheap tickets to Mexico City?"

"Let me look…"

The only really cheap ticket the agent can find leaves on Saturday and returns on Tuesday. It's Wednesday today.

"I'll take it."

I don't want to go for any longer than this anyway. There's only so far that even I can ignore the possibilities that loom when going to a country far away two weeks before a major operation that I am becoming more and more in need of. I chat away while he books the ticket, telling him how I've spontaneously decided to go alone and haven't told anyone. I *don't* tell him anything about my illness or pending operation. He's excited, like he's in on my secret.

"Make sure you come back and tell us how it went!"

I dip very heavily into the overdraft on my bank account, with the reasonable thought that if there is any time to feel no remorse about spending money I don't have, this is it. Once the ticket is booked, no one argues with me. Friends offer support, if reluctantly, as well as Spanish lessons and advice on where to stay. They have less than twenty-four hours to intervene, anyway. Blair accepts the inevitability of my journey.

When I visit my friend Dawn to tell her about it, I explain, "I think I'm going to die. They're going to put me under the anaesthetic for my surgery and they'll screw up and that's it. I won't wake up."

It's the first time I've said it out loud.

We're sitting on her balcony smoking menthol cigarettes and drinking sugary tea. I rarely smoke, and then not usually menthol, and I *never* put sugar in my tea. I am surprised at the yummy combination.

"You don't think you're going to die. You just love the drama of imagining your own funeral. And even if they did screw up, you wouldn't let them kill you anyway. You would refuse to die."

I like the analysis. I appreciate the confidence she has in my subconscious powers.

"You would be so mad you would will yourself to wake up to punish them."

But I still feel the two theories aren't mutually exclusive. Yes, I enjoy the drama of imagining my own funeral, but it is still a fear striking me to my core. They have the power to screw up and kill me. It's not impossible, and there's nothing I can do about it. As I pointed out in my first trip to the ER, no one expects to die suddenly. And my uncle's death imprinted this knowledge.

Years later, Dawn tells me that despite her casual acceptance of my news, she was horrified that I was going to Mexico. "I just thought, what can I say to Julie to convince her not to go? Nothing. If I tell her it's a terrible idea and I'm worried about her, she'll probably go for even longer just to prove she can."

I tell my mum that I'm going to Montreal to an anti-war conference with my friend Martine. I like the alliteration: Montreal with Martine, Mexico with me. Blair reluctantly drives me to the airport.

5. Pilgrimage to Frida

The plane lands. I put on my small backpack and find a cab. The driver takes me to the centre of the city, the Zocolo. Saturday afternoon: it's heaving with people, cars and market stalls. I have memorized all the Spanish I might need, with possible responses. I walk a few blocks to the hotel I have picked out in the guidebook. It's now a warehouse clothing store. I quickly find somewhere else to stay. I go to my room, unpack some of my things, and go out in search of groceries. Dry bread and bottled water are the safest route to digestive comfort. Walking back to the hotel, I see a sign that says, "Colon."

I'm shocked; I do a double take. It's a clothing store. Called "Colon." Two weeks before surgeons hack mine out. The store is just a block away from where I am staying.

I go back to my room and suddenly have no idea what to do. I am overwhelmed by a wave of complete helplessness. I sit on the bed and cry. Weep and shake. Gasp and choke. Clench my fists. Punch things. I am exactly as far away as I need to be to let go, to allow the rage, the sense of impotence to actually envelop me in a way that isn't just blank numbness. To stop "holding up" for everyone else.

I start drawing in my sketchbook. Colourful images of bloody colons and a violent self-portrait with the words "certain women bleed" scrawled across it. When I calm down I decide that I need to go out and be places where other people are. I get on a tour bus. It's dusk; the bus takes us all around the city until it is dark and the lights are twinkling. I realize that I'm not very lonely when I eavesdrop on several conversations and discover that I find myself more entertaining.

The next day is my pilgrimage to Frida. I remember the moment we met. It was a day of usual greyness and cold at my cold and grey university campus. I was going to the tutorial for my Intro to Women's Studies course in second-year undergrad. In an unusual turn of events, I actually got to the bookstore to buy the book we are supposed to be studying. I always had a very pragmatic approach to my degree. There was only a certain amount of information that I could retain and that my professors could ascertain whether I understood. I pledged to learn exactly that amount with minimal expense and little time spent. I was always involved in multiple activist campaigns, and usually at least a couple of jobs to pay my tuition, and so far this method had gotten me good marks. So I pick up this small book of Frida Kahlo's artwork and get to my class early. I start flipping through it, seeing her for the first time. My heart is in my throat, my stomach in my knees. "Moved" does not aptly describe my response. Every cell of my being is shaken. I want to know everything. Who she is and where these paintings came from. I read about her life, her sickness, her revolutionary struggles—political and personal. I am bursting.

The class starts, and the teaching assistant, Sarah, enthusiastically asks us what we think of the art. She is met by a torrent of groans. "I don't get it." "It's gross." The comments make me so angry that I explode. Little bloody bits of Julie all over the tutorial space, all in aid of a dead artist whom I feel like I have just met. After this, whenever I hear of exhibits of her art within driving distance I go to see them. When the Hollywood film comes out, I don't want to see it until several people I trust assure me that it's actually good. When I watch it, I want to be there, inside. And now I am.

I think the point of travel is less about the moment I inhabit a space and more about creating different rooms in my head. The more places I visit physically, the more places there are to escape to mentally. I want to feel Frida's room so I can go back whenever I want to — co-opting real places to form imaginary spaces in my body, like a giant mansion I can wander through at leisure.

So it's Sunday. The day is bright and warm. I take the public transit out to Coyoacan and walk to her house. I don't anticipate how right I am to take this trip until I am standing there, in the courtyard of the Blue House. I take out my sketchbook and sit there, drawing for hours. I go through the house where the paintings are hung, lingering at each one. I stand in her bedroom. Looking at the clock stopped above her bed. It's twenty-two minutes past nine in Frida's room.

I think there's an element to the way our lives are lived as women that makes it easier to tear the scabs off — to reveal things about the world, about oppression. Some critics have described Frida's work as self-absorbed and apolitical. Frida herself wanted to create art that would have more "use" politically, a self-conscious perspective that I can relate to. It's hard not to feel this pull, this judgment, when undertaking works that are so violently personal. She used political expression to heal her medical wounds. I have an imaginary critic in my head who describes my work as "the vapid rantings of post-adolescent womanhood." I prefer to believe that a single story can say something broader about the worlds we live in.

I buy a hand-embroidered blanket from a man on the street, a few blocks from Frida's house. Bright, beautiful colours. I decide to give it to my former hospital roommate, Ali, who I have just heard is back in the hospital. I walk to Trotsky's house. I look at his study, his books, his typewriter. I touch his stove when nobody's looking. I go back and walk through the parks, the markets. I get on a bus that seems to be going to San Angel, but it ends its route in a place that looks very far from the Diego Rivera Museum on the map. I stop and ask an older couple, in my appallingly bad Spanish, how I should get there. Before I even know what's happening the man of the couple is hailing down a bus and having an animated conversation with the driver. Lots of hand waving is going on, and I can't make out what is being said. He pays the driver and turns to me. He points to a spot on the map that is very close to the museum and says, "He'll take you there. You just have to walk a little bit."

I try to pay him back, but he declines. "No, no, have fun!"

The Rivera Museum is the home and studio that Diego designed for him and Frida in their later years. The studios and living quarters are separate, one side for her, one for him, with a bridge connecting them in the middle.

I get to the entrance an hour before the museum is scheduled to close.

A security guard stops me at the door and explains something in Spanish. I really don't understand what he's saying but figure out from his gesturing that there are film crews inside and they have closed early for these people.

I keep pointing at my watch and pleading with my eyes.

"Por favor, por favor... Solo uno momento."

I don't really care if the words are fitting together properly because he starts smiling and sneaks me in. The people rushing around with their cameras are all North American and speaking English, so I really don't care that they're giving me death looks for interrupting their work. I have not come from Toronto to be kept out of Frida's studio by pretentious film students. When I leave, I sit across the street for a couple of hours, sketching the outside of the studio, bathing in the warm Mexican sun and drinking it all in. I walk up to the subway station and go back to my hotel. Tired, at peace, I fall asleep. The next day, I go up the tower to look at the whole city. I write postcards, postcards, and more postcards. The physical and temporal distance from home provides perspective. The farther I move physically from the scene, the greater vision I have of its entire face and content. I can more accurately assess the size and significance of the individual elements in relation to one another.

In the afternoon, I sit on the steps of the Palacio Nacional trying to absorb the scope of Rivera's mural of Mexican history. I am feeling a bit starved for human contact because my broken Spanish is seriously inhibitive to meaningful dialogue. An Australian couple gets to the top of the steps and flop down. I listen to their conversation for a while before deciding that they are people I want to talk to. So I do, and we get along right away.

We decide to go out for dinner. It is the first time I actually indulge in Mexican cuisine, but seeing as it's my last night, I am daring enough to stray from my bread and bottled water digestive safety diet. We order several dishes to share and giant Sangrias. The food is bliss. They walk me back to my hotel. It is pouring rain, so I suggest that we go to a nearby cafe until it lets up. When we get inside, we realize that the cafe is actually a giant, ancient-looking courtyard. A beautiful concrete structure that has been converted into a hot nightclub at weekends and a trendy cafe on weeknights. The environment is dreamlike—we're sitting in an ancient place in the middle of Mexico City where the staff are playing the new Radiohead album.

I start drifting away with Thom Yorke's ethereal voice. In the corner, I see Frida sitting with her sister Christina and Diego. She looks at me, eyes twinkling, and invites me over. I have to push and elbow my way through a crowd of art student ghosts who even in the metaphysical world are trying to get close to her.

We sit and drink and watch the rain let up. A thick fog descends, and I suddenly feel lighter, more transparent, as if I could float. I turn to Frida. "You know, I always imagine you in my revolutionary army. When I can't bear the thought of going into a situation alone, I pretend that you're there with all the people I know would have my back, marching en masse behind me."

She smiles. "I know."

I want to issue a formal invitation. "Frida, will you really be in my army?"

She cups her hand under my chin, her fingers on my cheek. "Jules, you know I'm already there."

Her smile lights me through to my core. Later, as I walk out alone into the fog and back to my hotel, I realize that neither of us had accents, and I can't really even remember the words we said. I guess that's what happens when souls speak.

Back in my hotel room, I don't mind the all-night trips back and forth to the washroom from the spicy Mexican food and alcohol. Deking out the cockroaches isn't really a problem either. The advantage to tropical bugs is that you can hear them coming, giant scuttling things. The mosquitoes focus on my inflamed joints — they have clever little noses, with the power to sense where all the hot rushing blood has collected.

6. Trillium Welfare Queen

After Mexico, all I have to do is wait. I am frustrated, terrified, but I am continually told by everyone how well I am dealing with it all. The truth is, I don't know what else to do. How to *not* cope. There are just so many details that I have to remain on top of. I've been dealing with Trillium, the provincial government program that reimburses people with low incomes who have high prescription drug costs. I am officially almost a no-income person at this point, making bits of money on short-term contracts and part-time work, but mostly living off Blair and my parents.

It is an absurdly bureaucratic process, requiring all kinds of obscure documentation. Although I was approved months ago, I am constantly having my claims returned. Trillium has refused to accept the statement from my insurance company that I exceeded my coverage halfway through the year. They need a letter addressed to them. So I phone the insurance company. I leave a message asking for the letter. It doesn't come. So I phone back and leave another message. No return phone call. No letter. When I phone again, I finally speak to a human being.

"Well, I can't write you a letter that isn't true."

Her tone betrays a certain pride in having caught me red-handed in my attempts to defraud the system. As if I've found some kind of secret, recreational purpose for colitis treatments. *'Cuz steroid enemas are street, yo.*

Now I am the Trillium Drug Plan Welfare Queen.

"I'm not asking you to. My coverage ran out in January."

"No, no, it didn't. I have it right here. You were reimbursed for receipts dated in March."

I have meticulously filed all correspondence from the insurance company. I pull out the record she is referring to and immediately see the problem.

"I submitted all of my receipts together, and you didn't reimburse them in order. So I have a stack of receipts from January and February that were not reimbursed and two from March that were."

"That's impossible. The computer wouldn't do that."

"Well, here's the record number. It should be on my file, and it will tell you that it did."

She types the number into the computer and aggressively replies, "Well, I don't know why it did that."

She agrees to write the letter.

So this is what my life has become. Begging for money for agonizing treatments I didn't even want to take and that completely failed to work. What if I was too ill to deal with these details? Most people who need the plan are too sick to deal with the roadblocks designed into it. How many seniors on multiple medications have the capacity to file and analyze every piece of paper that comes in the mail? A taste for what friends of mine in the States have described happens with every medical bill—HMOs fighting for every payment. It seems so obvious to me that this is what happens when for-profit insurance companies are in charge.

I go online and curiously start poking around insurance rate sheets from US companies to assess the cost of my treatments. It's possible that having a unionized carpenter, first, for a father and, now, for a husband means that my health care benefits would be good. But who knows. It's also possible that me and my problem colon would be uninsurable. So adding up the costs from spring 2002 to fall 2003, I exceed half a million dollars before I get too depressed and stop adding. My mum comes in while I'm doing this and suggests that I add the hours I've spent negotiating medical and university bureaucracies as a result of my illness.

"Make sure you charge consulting rates!" she says. "Not just your normal hourly wage."

We laugh because in reality my time as a sick person is not valuable enough that anyone would even consider covering the cost of it. With every encroachment from the cold bureaucracies of everyday life, the warmth of the Mexican sun fades from my skin.

7. Willow the Brat Cat

One night, I'm showing my Mexico pictures to Martine, the friend who I told my mum I was in Montreal with. While I was gone, she had been involved in a kitty rescue. A house in her neighbourhood was overrun with cats and Martine decided to adopt just one. When she went to pick him up, a second kitten started demanding her attention. She was a scrawny little white fluffball, following Martine around and saying, "Myahh! Myahiih! Myahh!"

The little kitten was relentless. She was the only survivor from her litter and clearly had a strategy. Martine took both kittens home to her partner, and they named the little white one Other Julie. I didn't get that they named her *after* me. I thought they just named her that as a way of enticing me to adopt her because they really just wanted to keep the first kitten. So I tell them I want her and I rename her Willow Rosenberg, after the *Buffy* character. It's not until months later, when I'm with Martine explaining to someone else how Martine got me to take the kitten, that she tells me. "No, we wanted her. We named her Other Julie because, well, how can I put this. She followed me around yakking and yakking and she kept doing tricks and funny things until we paid attention to her. She was a card. And, well, a brat. So we said, 'Look, it's Julie!' And that's how she got her name."

8. *Basta! Basta! Basta!*

The next scene begins, as all health care encounters do, in the waiting room.

As I enter the hospital, the music from my iPod floods out all hospital sensation, drowning out my anxiety—Asian Dub Foundation blasting political sentiment that exactly echoes my feelings about the medical establishment, the illness, my colon—"*Basta! Basta! Basta!*" Enough, enough, enough. I'm not allowed to have anyone with me because we're still in the SARS scare in Toronto and only people with appointments are allowed in the hospital.

I'm feeling emboldened, confident, and...terrified. A nurse greets me. "You can just sit right over here."

She leads me to an examining table in a room where there is scope equipment looming about threateningly. I can feel the machines and hoses looking at me. I try to stare them down, but there are too many of them and they are just too powerful. After several years of colitis and endless painful scopes of my very inflamed and bleeding bowels, I can't even look at the machines when they're off.

I venture into the hall to find a trashy magazine to bring back to the room. I'm still waiting forty minutes after the time my appointment is scheduled for. Shania Twain is on the radio. I consider the possibility that in my weakened, vulnerable state, my pretensions may fade away long enough to find some innocent enjoyment in "Man! I Feel Like a Woman." No such luck. The intensity of the cringe just increases. Coolness is such a curse.

I pick up a pamphlet about the surgery I'm going to have—the one about sex. It is all about having an "understanding" partner and suggesting that I should not worry if I do not feel like having sex for three or four months after the surgery. I'm terrified by this random, unsubstantiated statistic. I am overwhelmed by my desire to be desired, to have my sexuality acknowledged. There is no discussion of why a bowel surgery would have this drastic libidinal impact.

Enter the young Dr. Leonard—a medical resident and surgeon-in-training, sent to educate me about my pending operation. He's one of the nice ones. Matter-of-factly describing the surgery, what happens afterwards, the drugs, the cutting, the next surgery, the...

But me, all I want to know is, *Will I be sexy? Am I SEXY?* And the annoying thing is that I don't think he's sexy. He's not bad, but it's not like I'm fantasizing about jumping the doctor. So I ask about drugs and milligrams and adrenal glands and amphetamines and steroid withdrawal depression...

Like depression—don't you get it?... Will I be SEXY? But if there's one person in the world who certainly won't answer my internal dialogue, it's someone who's gone through medical training. They rarely deign to answer explicit questions. So I thank him for the information, and he nods, appearing grateful that I don't have any more questions.

He then directs me to the office of Kathy, the stoma nurse, about ten floors above the surgeon's. Kathy's job is to pick the best spot for the bag, the external appliance that will hold my stool after the surgery. She has cartoons about stomas on her door. She wants to draw the spot where my intestine will be pulled out of my stomach and into the bag with a green marker.

"So have you thought about where you want it?"

She makes me sit with my steroid-cushioned, colitis-bloated tummy hanging out of my pants. She pokes and asks. Forwards and backwards.

"It needs to sit on top," she says.

I picture skinny girls with no top on, and she says, "Do you know where you want it?"

And I say, "I *don't* want it."

And she says, "I know. Here's my card. Call me if you want to talk about it."

And I say, "I don't want to talk and I'm not going to think about it until it's there and then I'll pretend that it's not there."

And she says, "That's okay, that's one way to deal, but call me if you change your mind."

I don't. Instead I meet a friend in a bar and drink some rum. It doesn't help.

A week later, it's time for the scope. When I arrive, they take me into the room with all the gurneys. A nurse starts my IV and wheels me into the room with the machines. The surgeon comes in to see me. "So we've got your surgery scheduled for next week."

I notice the smell of the Body Shop perfume White Musk. I ask the nurse if that's what she's wearing. It is. I appreciate the comfort of pleasant fragrance instead of the usual hospital fare. Then Dr. Leonard, the resident who I met at my "education" appointment, starts talking to me and administering my meds in such a way that I realize that *he* is going to perform the scope. The resident. Not Athena the gentle surgeon. But I feel too weak and helpless to argue.

"Do you have your period?" The nurse motions toward the string attached to my tampon, dangling between my legs.

I want to say, *Nope, I just think tampons are fun.* But I answer honestly. "Yes, why? Should I not be wearing a tampon?"

It did occur to me that it might be a problem but I wanted to be clean and smell nice, so I put it in before I bathed in lavender bath salts that morning.

"Well, it would be better if you weren't; it could make it more difficult to scope you, but that's okay."

"I'll just take it out then." I reach between my legs and pull it out.

The nurse looks shocked. Dr. Leonard quickly averts his eyes as if to give me privacy and, frankly, looks somewhat horrified. The nurse rushes to find me something sterile to put it in and padding to put underneath me in case I bleed. Apparently, I should be more squeamish about admitting that I menstruate when I lie naked in front of a room of medical professionals. I do not claim to understand their reasoning.

I am still puzzling over this when he starts.

I gasp. "The medication is not working. It's really hurting!"

The White Musk Nurse says, "But he's not doing anything right now."

As if I have some kind of investment in lying about the fact that the camera with the hose jammed into my body still hurts, whether or not he is actively pushing it at that exact moment.

Athena comes back and tells him to stop.

He protests, "But we hardly got anywhere."

He looks at me accusingly and says with disappointment, "There's hardly anything there." Meaning disease, I presume.

I am frustrated because obviously on the dose of steroids I am taking, the symptoms are *masked*. We know this.

And then Athena looks at me. She shrugs and smiles. "I just needed to see how bad the disease was." And she leaves.

I think about how medical science has methods and orders that must have some kind of general rationale, but when they don't make sense in the moment, I feel like logic is ultimately subsumed by the importance of rigid traditions. And education. So the resident learned something. I'm not entirely clear on what—I just know it wasn't what I would have taught him. A lesson on scoping the body—as if I were a landmass to be explored, mapped out, by cartographers of human flesh.

What I learn is even more profound. The surgical resident is scared of my vagina. The idea of an actively menstruating woman replacing the disembodied anus, rectum, and colon he's focused on is terrifying to him.

9. The Grand Cutting

There are many Julies.

One is sitting at her computer writing this story, Iron and Wine providing the soundtrack, with street noise and the voices of playing children floating through my open window. My chocolate mint herb plant winds onto my computer, combining scents with my beeswax candle and the burned sage in my prayer bowl. My dog sprawls at my feet as the cats alternate between meowing at the window to go out and meowing from the garden to come back in.

At the same time, there is another Julie, still lying on the table in the operating theatre, and yet another one, curled up in her hospital bed, knees tightly clutched to her chest, tears silently streaming down her face, raging, writing this next scene. I'm reaching through time right now to tell them that we're still here. We're all right.

So they're pushing me into the OR on a stretcher, and I say, "This is weird, this is so weird."

And the nurse says, "What's so weird about it?"

And I wonder if she can see that it's weirder than the spaceship on the *X-Files* where Scully had her chip inserted — with shining bright spotlights and TV cameras and screens and men in masks. I tell the man, the doctor, the anaesthesiologist, that he's not going to find a vein in my dehydrated hand after two days of me not eating, shitting liquid for the surgery prep to clean the intestine that they're about to hack out. Blair's adage, to never break a clean dish, occurs to me, but I guess dishwasher laws don't apply to surgeons.

So I tell him, "Here...in the crook of the elbow. You can't see the vein, but it's a good one. Go straight, go deep."

But he ignores me, as he steadfastly digs into my wrist bone with his needle. To distract myself, I turn my head and concentrate on the conversation about the colon, and what they're going to do with it, happening between the intern and the doctor four feet away. And I turn back in surprise as I feel the needle finally give up on the wrist and dig in deep in the crook of my elbow, good and straight, into the vein.

And he tells me that we're "in luck."

And I lose my temper and yell, "Lucky? Who's lucky?"

And he says, "Us. Lucky that we found any vein in you that we could put an IV in." And I pray for his fragile ego, so weak that he needs to lie when we both know he's lying.

And then the nurse leans in and says, "My name's Marla. I have colitis. I know how you're feeling." Angel nurse.

And Needle Guy starts yelling about antibiotics and something and finally says, "Well, fine, I won't give her any then!"

And I look up at Angel Nurse and say, "I'm not going into this surgery without antibiotics."

And she says, "No, you're not. He's grumpy; he's venting. You're going to get antibiotics." She's livid. "It's uncalled for! Nobody should be speaking like this while you're awake." And she looks up at him and says, "While the patient's awake!"

And as he injects my "lucky" IV line with sedatives, I feel my mouth open and hear words I might have repressed coming out with rage. "And you know what else is uncalled for? People talking about my colon like

I'm not even here and saying 'it' and 'the' like it's no big deal, but it's my colon and it's a really big deal!"

And Angel Nurse says, "It is. It is a really big deal."

And I like to think that at this point the frog-faced-mask-, hat-, scrubs-wearing doctors move slightly backwards, but I can't be sure if they recoil at the vague realization of how horrific they are being with the almost naked human-butcher project lying like a slab on narrow metal because Angel Nurse and Tantrum Doctor are leaning over me and saying, "Okay, Julie, you're going under. Keep your eyes open, your eyes open."

And I try and try, and then I am gone. And everyone who said you don't dream under anaesthetic is wrong.

I'm on a shoreline. It's familiar but I just can't place it. I'm walking somewhere with purpose, I just don't know where. I drift into other dreams. I dream of a world where health care is fully funded and where med students are taught manners. I dream of a world where sick people are comforted, where our feet are massaged with lavender oil as trays of sweet-smelling organic foods are brought to us in bed. I dream of health care that's about *healing*. And of healers who acknowledge and respect me as a whole — intellectual, emotional, sexual, spiritual — woman. I dream of hospital pyjamas that cover our entire bodies in comfortable fabrics and pleasant colours. And slippers. I dream of slippers.

Before I go under, I try to determine what kind of accent Needle-guy has. Now, it's the first voice I hear in the recovery room. "Julie, Julie…"

"Are you Italian?" I ask him. I feel like I am glowing. I'm so relieved to wake up from the surgery I'm giddy. I'm also really well medicated.

"No," he says. "I'm Bulgarian."

"That's okay!" I say brightly. I wave my hands in the air. "*Molto grazie!*"

I have forgiven him for his lack of social skills, I am just intensely grateful that he got me through the surgery without incident. My three biggest fears — waking up while they're still cutting, being half-awake and bored for hours, and/or dying — have all been quelled.

He laughs appreciatively and I can hear him at the nurses' station as he leaves the room — "And then I said, 'No, I'm Bulgarian,' and she said, 'That's okay. *Molto grazie!*'"

They laugh uproariously as I ponder my curious urge to speak Italian. A nurse comes to talk to me. "Hi, I'm Doris," she says.

"Hi, how did it go? I want to know everything. Did it go well? Did they do it all laparoscopically or did they have to cut? Tell me everything!"

She laughs, looking up at another nurse, smiling. "She wants to know everything." And to me, "Yes, it went very well. The entire surgery was laparoscopic; you're doing really well."

"Can you put your hand on my shoulder, please? I just feel so, so weird."

She complies, rubbing my arm comfortingly. I ask her about her day. She tells me a funny story about her cat, Harry Houdini, who refuses to use litter boxes, so she has to take him for walks before she goes to work. I tell her about my cat, Willow Rosenberg, named after the character on *Buffy*. We agree that self-determination for cats is important. They deserve their own last names.

She decides that she wants to take me up to my room herself.

As she pushes me into my room where my mum and Blair wait, I sit up cheerfully and introduce her, "This is Doris. She's super!"

I put a picture of our wedding on my bedside table. When the nurses continue to talk to me like I'm five, I say emphatically, "I'm twenty-four. Look at my wedding picture!" The irony of this is that I remember actually turning five and thinking, *Finally, people will stop talking to me like a little kid.* And then, when they continued to talk down to me I'd think defiantly, *Don't they know I'm five?* Blair buys me a gorgeous reproduction of Frida's *Self-Portrait in Frame* for my wall, and my windowsill and trays are covered in cards, baskets, and flowers from well-wishers.

The next morning, the stoma nurse is at my bedside. It is now one day after The Grand Cutting. She wants me to learn how to change the bag and use it, but I can't look. She removes the bag that is adhered to my lower-right abdomen and cleanses it and talks to me.

"Don't you know that there's no nerve endings in a stoma?"

But I can feel every touch, every movement. The inside of my body is now on the outside, and I want to throw up.

Having successfully staved off entreaties from health care professionals encouraging me to acquaint myself with my new abdominal terrain, I concentrate very, very hard on the TV. I have an addiction to all-news stations, but predictably wars and violence are making me incredibly anxious. So for safety I retreat into the set of *The Ellen DeGeneres Show,* finding refuge in what appears in my morphine-induced, post-surgical haze to be Ellen's golden halo. I'm not sure if it's just the drugs or if it's also the desperation for something comfortable, something happy, but Ellen is glowing. She's grinning from ear to ear, and I'm transported into her welcoming, comfortable surroundings. I'm sitting in the constructed living room of her show, laughing along with her and her celebrity guests. I'm dancing in the audience. I'm anywhere but here, in the bleakness of this post-surgical recovery. As the day progresses, I continue pushing the button on the morphine pump. It's the most drugs I've ever had, and I feel slightly disconnected, not present in the world of IV poles and ileostomy bags. At one point, I'm watching the news, and I don't notice for about fifteen minutes in that it's actually in Italian. This is strange. Despite the fact my mum is Italian, we never speak it at home, and my fluency is sketchy at best. Has the morphine unlocked the language comprehension part of my brain? Or am I hallucinating a different broadcast in English? I'll never know.

A nurse comes in to drain the bag at the end of the catheter inserted into my urethra. She looks alarmed. "Uh-oh, it's not draining properly."

"What do you mean?" I ask. "Do I have to pee to fill the bag up?"

"No," she replies in the same ridiculing tone that everyone I asked the same question last night used. "Your bladder should just be drained by the catheter. You don't even feel it."

It quickly turns into the classic input-output question. Apparently, they have put lots of liquid in through the IV and nothing is coming out of the catheter. She moves quickly to page someone, telling me, "Your bladder might have been punctured during the surgery; it might be leaking into the rest of your body."

I don't believe her. I feel pretty sure that my bladder is full and I just really, really need to pee.

"Just let me try and pee. I've probably been holding it because it would be really weird to pee in bed."

She looks vaguely amused but mostly annoyed. She answers plainly. "That's impossible."

I release my bladder muscles and immediately flood the catheter tubing, filling up the bag with 800 cc's. Her eyes widen as the bag gets fuller and fuller. I smile triumphantly.

"See, I was holding it."

She huffs. "Well, they must have put it in wrong then."

Which makes no sense to me at all. I can clearly feel myself either holding my pee or releasing it to rush through the tube. Her objection seems to be an apt metaphor for my hospitalization. Health care professionals who feel that they must control everything so they must deny and crush my muscular resistance. No one ever comes to see whether the catheter has in fact been "put in wrong."

Joanne is amply impressed when I tell her about my ability to control the catheter. I explain, "So I'm lying here, thinking, I really, really feel like I need to pee. But I'm in bed. So I hold it…"

"Like you do," she cuts in.

I laugh. "Exactly. Who pees in bed? But it turns out, I *can* hold it. Even with the tube in. They can't figure it out."

"Wow, you already have a party trick."

My sister calls from New York, where she has just started her PhD. Our phone call is repeatedly interrupted by the arrival of my new loud and whiny roommate, Marni, who keeps picking up the phone and hanging up again really loudly. She screams and moans and whines at every single thing the doctors and nurses do: from taking blood, to injections, to moving at all. She has no concept of "medium volume" in her speech, much less speaking quietly at 2:30 a.m. when I've finally fallen asleep. She had surgery three days before me, but really wants to play up the pain she's going through to get more attention and sympathy. Obviously, I don't mind people expressing pain to medical professionals; I guess I just feel like we patients need a common strategy. Screaming blue murder about having your vitals taken is the sort of thing that makes the rest of us lose credibility.

Rounds happen at 6:00 a.m. every morning. I still haven't actually worked up the courage to look at my ileostomy bag yet. It's clear, so my inflamed and bloody stoma is visible. Five med students and a doctor gather around my bed. The junior resident does all the talking, with a forced air of authority and confidence. I am kind of hazy, but compliant when they ask to see my abdomen. It's the kind of question that really only has the question mark at the end to produce some kind of vague air of obtaining consent.

"Would you mind lifting your gown up? Do you mind if we take a look?"

I lie here, on display, the Live Art Sub-total Colectomy with End-Ileostomy Exhibition. I look up at them to avoid looking at the bag, and see two of the students whispering to one another, clearly engrossed in a separate conversation.

Am I boring you? Sorry, would you like me to strip a little more? I am tempted to say it, but too hazy to deal with the potential fallout, so I restrain myself. I also notice that they shaved off my pubic hair. I can't figure out why they would have done this; it's some distance from all the incisions and they didn't shave anywhere near the tubes they inserted. I find this profoundly annoying because I rarely shave anywhere, much less extremely sensitive areas that grow back with ingrown hairs and painful, itchy bumps. I am flooded with embarrassment and horror imagining the scene when they looked down at my sheeted body on the operating table and decided that the bush needed to go. If they warned me at the pre-op appointment that I would have to look pre-pubescent to proceed with the surgery, I would have waxed it all off for them.

"Great, looks great!" the junior resident says.

But my actual state is reflected more accurately in the eyes of the students who are incapable or unwilling to disguise their disgust. They all leave.

The morphine pump makes me so itchy that I'm scratching patches of skin off, leaving a rash covering most of my body. It also makes the words on the page swim and even the most vacuous of TV shows difficult to understand. To drown out my princess-roommate's snoring at night I put on headphones and listen to the TV. I figure the news will put me to sleep, so I leave it on CNN. But I'm on such large doses of steroids that no amount of morphine lets me sleep properly. CNN leads to fevered dreams about wars and bombings and George W. is talking and I'm sure he is in the room somewhere.

"Julie!" The floating George Bush head smiles vacantly at me.

"Ahhh! Go away!" I scream in terror.

Bush-Head grins and whispers, "Weapons of Mass Destruction. Liberation. Torture."

I shudder, yanking off my earphones and turning off the news. I stop pushing the morphine button and eventually rock myself to sleep.

The next morning, my stoma bag is full to overflowing. Gaseous and painful. The nurse is young. Very young and pretty with lots of eyeliner. She promises to come back and help, but she doesn't.

It's heavy and it hurts.

Blair goes to the nurses' station. "Where's her nurse? She needs a nurse!"

And they say, "She's on her lunch. It'll be half an hour."

No one is covering for her.

But I can't wait.

"Ask him," I tell Blair, pointing at Ulysses, the nurse my evil roommate from hell has running back and forth at her beck and call.

Ulysses responds by yelling impatiently from across the room, "What can I help you with?"

And I say, "Can you just come here when you have a minute?" So he comes, and I say, "I need help, I don't know how to change it. It hurts."

He looks at me like I'm disgusting, definitely not sexy, and says, "Okay, okay, I'll come back."

He doesn't.

Another nurse comes and says, "Okay, let's go to the bathroom."

She leads me to the toilet and says, "Okay, sit down."

And I say, "On the toilet? With my pants down?"

And she looks at me and says, "Yes."

So I do it. With my belly and the smelly bag hanging. She's thin, but at least she's not pretty. And the bag falls. Splats on the floor and liquid shit and green bile are everywhere and she says it's okay, but it's not.

She hands me toilet paper and tells me to hold the stoma. It's the first time I've seen it. It's red and bloody and violently sputtering and protruding from my perfect, smooth, cream belly, and I cry. I cry and I cry and I tell her that I can't look, and she rhythmically responds as she wipes and cleanses, wipes and cleans, and says that it's normal and that everything I'm feeling and all the emotions are normal and fine and she rinses and deodorizes the smelly plastic bag to the rhythm of my tears, but it's not normal. I'm sitting on a toilet with my legs wide open with a red piece of my small intestine hanging and—did I mention?—*sputtering*. Nothing is normal. I want to throw up.

10. The Shower Scene

I desperately want a shower. I am not allowed and not physically able to go by myself, but I don't want to ask a nurse. So I ask Blair to take me. I am feeling very ambivalent about this. The idea of being naked alone with my partner and washing the hospital film off of my skin is very appealing. It is also terrifying. I wonder if he will be disgusted with my ileostomy bag that is in hospital-regulation clear plastic to make my "output" visible for professional monitoring. I am frightened that he will find me sexually repellent. As we stand in the hospital shower, I tell him my fears.

He looks at me very intently and says, "The bag is just something on you. It's not you. You're still sexy, you're still Julie."

We later joke that I should alter the educational brochure to reflect that my desire for sexual contact was dampened for about three or four hours after surgery rather than three or four months.

II. Naked Onstage

Now I'm onstage. Re-enacting this moment four years later. Being topless in a public theatre to perform this hospital shower scene is much less frightening than lying prone in an operating theatre. I have been performing "tamer" aspects of the show and remaining clothed for the past year, so this moment is a breakthrough for me.

My friend Loree Erickson is organizing a cabaret about disability and sexuality, and at first, when she invites me to perform, I'm not sure why. I'm thrilled and immediately say yes, but at this point, nothing I've performed has been remotely about sex. It's true that I start by taking my clothes off and putting on a hospital gown. But this striptease joke was a way of saying that health care encounters are *always* intimate. On some level, medical training acknowledges this intimacy by how intensely it attempts to erase notions of sensuality and sexuality. The cold, biomedical mapping procedures remove any evocation of flesh. Everything about the way we are dressed in hospital gowns and scrubs, and the stiff and formal ways we are expected to relate, are designed to repress any overt sexual overtone in this highly intimate encounter. From where I lie, all of this effort at de-sexualization reveals profound fears about what happens to, and between, all of our bodies every time flesh touches flesh. By taking off my clothes publicly in a non-hospital environment I was demonstrating my vulnerability on my own terms. Considering I'd mostly performed for academic audiences, it was a fun way to shake up the format of the typical conference paper that I couldn't bring myself to give anymore.

So the first thing that occurs to me when preparing this performance is that I want to get way more naked than I have in my regular venues. Loree's own work about sex is so cutting-edge and groundbreaking that, just from seeing it, I feel this new wave of confidence about what I could actually do onstage. In all of my early trips to emergency departments and doctor's offices, I was very compliant with the command to take off everything but my underwear and put the gown on. And then I start thinking about the fact that I did *write* about sex, even if I didn't perform about it. I include the scenes from my manuscript where I pull out my tampon, where I internally agonize about my sexiness with the resident, and where Blair honours my post-surgical body in the hospital shower.

It's so important to me to reveal more than just my medical vulnerability. I want to be visible and strong and sexual in my body too. Leakiness is more than weakness. Acknowledging that we're not the contained and separate beings we're supposed to be — but are actually leaking and flowing into each other all the time — is powerful to me. It's the first time I perform the scene where I wake up from dreams about CNN reports and start yelling at the floating Bush-Head. There were news reports about him having a colonoscopy the day before and the timing is just too good. I can't resist telling the activist crowd who have so beautifully witnessed my pain, trauma, and vulnerability, "Did anyone else hear that George Bush had a colonoscopy yesterday? This makes me happy."

The crowd bursts out laughing and cheers at the cheeky but enjoyable possibility that a world leader may also have endured some kind of similar suffering. When I get off this stage, I'm so grateful to Loree and her awesome community for creating such a safe space for me to be naked in — to bring out the pieces of the story that are the most vulnerable and terrifying for me to expose. Blair is standing at the bottom of the stairs, tears streaming down his face. I'm kind of shocked; this is the first time through any of the illnesses or performances about illness that he's cried. He pulls me into a tight hug, his wet face shaking against my neck. I can't remember what he says here. Whatever it is, I'm not sure what to say back. His uncharacteristic tearfulness has drawn out something equally uncharacteristic in me — utter speechlessness.

The next day, I am interviewed for *Chatelaine* magazine. It's a fantasy coming true. Over a sushi lunch, I talk about my illness, my work, my hopes for the future of medicine. When the magazine is published, I get a massive response on the *My Leaky Body* website and am invited to perform and facilitate workshops across the country for the next year. So here I become Miss Chatelaine. Obviously, this title is steeped in irony like well-brewed ironic tea. And, yes, I know that stating this defeats the purpose of being ironic, but I couldn't risk a redux of the grade eleven drama class when I stuffed my bra to play a failed beauty queen because it was funny and the boys at the back of the class thought I was really pretending my breasts had grown exponentially overnight and that they "figured it out" that my new bosom was just sweat socks.

The funniest part for me is when Blair goes to work and shows all the guys that his wife is in *Chatelaine*. Someone he doesn't know very well doesn't believe him and is all like, "Yeah, right. That's not your wife."

Blair gets home and tells me and I can't stop laughing. I mean if you're going to pick a fake wife from a magazine to show off to your construction worker buddies, pick the blonde on the cover. Not the one on page twenty-three in the hospital gown. But whatever. The point is, I'm not Miss Chatelaine, and yet, I *so* was. I get emails from patients and family members and health care workers who identify with my experience, and lots of requests for tickets for the next performance in Toronto.

Around the same time, Blair and I have moved into a new house, and a short walk away, an amazing new business called Red Tent Sisters has just opened up. Two young women, Kim and Amy Sedgwick, started this store and wellness centre, entirely dedicated to nurturing and celebrating women's bodies and health. I rent the same space Loree held her cabaret in and do a three-night run to audiences I mostly don't recognize. Dawn directs the show with the support of some awesome theatre people I've recently met. And she single-handedly runs the house while Blair manages the stage. Red Tent Sisters sponsors these shows, setting up tables at the theatre and advertising the shows in their store. Although I feel nervous in the days before I perform, it's such an amazing gift to have so many people around to support me. As soon as I step onto the stage and look into the eyes of the audience who have come to hear my stories, my nerves wash away. And then some part of this future me that confidently performs these tales on stage reaches back and bends the strings of time to whisper in the ear of the Julie enduring the trauma years before.

12. Cheshire Cat Resident

Back in the post-surgical malaise of 2003, it's time for 6:00 a.m. rounds again. Same group. This time I realize that the doctor to my left is the one who casually discussed my colon with the student in the OR. What's more, the same student is standing at the foot of my bed, and he's also the one who was whispering to his friend behind their charts the day before. The junior resident, as usual, looks like the cat that has eaten the canary. Perhaps it's unfair, but I take his perpetual cheer as a patronizing affront.

"All right, well, we'll get you off this catheter so we can get you up and moving around! We've got to get you up and moving!"

I actually do want the catheter out and have already been up and moving around. And while I maintain an air of remarkable ease, it does seriously hurt. It feels like someone has tied my belly button to the back of my ribs and pumped my stomach with a gas station tire inflator.

I also just want to fight.

"Well, that's fine. As long as you know that I'm going to be pushing my morphine button a lot more because it really hurts to move. And I don't really see the point anyway. Why can't I just keep the catheter and I'll move around anyway?"

He maintains his painted Cheshire Cat grin.

"Well, I guess you can keep it until this afternoon then, but we want to get you up and moving around!"

He uses his "and that's final, young lady" school-principal sort of tone as he moves away from the bed, clearly thinking he is being very generous with his compromise.

They all start to leave when I say, "Wait!"

They look back impatiently.

"I want to know what happened. No one has really told me what was done yet. What are all these incisions? Where did they go in? What exactly was cut and where, and what was left, and where are the internal sites?"

The other reason I stopped pushing the morphine button was because I actually wanted to feel what was going on in my body. I was tired of feeling like a slab of meat, numb, and completely at the whim of other people.

With his back still to me, he looks over his shoulder.

"Piece of cake!" he says inexplicably, with enthusiasm.

I look around, one eyebrow furiously about to break through the furrows in my forehead. I settle on the actual doctor, wondering if it is just me or if the resident is making no sense at all.

The resident chimes in again. "Those incisions will heal up in no time; you won't even feel it! Piece of cake!"

The doctor, possibly remembering my outburst on the operating table, quickly intervenes. "I was in on your operation. I'll tell you everything."

I wonder if he thinks I don't recognize him, that scrubs maintained his anonymity or that the anaesthetic erased the moments immediately preceding the operation from my memory.

"It's okay, you can go now." He shoos the students off.

He sits down on my bed and describes every detail. Where the cameras were, what tools were used. Exactly where they cut my sigmoid colon, what was left. What they had been able to see of the disease. I'm very impressed that my colon was taken out through my belly button. That three tiny keyhole scars, a stoma, and a line over my belly button is all that is left as evidence.

He explains that my colon is being biopsied and that the pathology reports will reveal the details of my actual diagnosis.

"But I've had lots of biopsies done," I tell him. "We *know* it's ulcerative colitis."

"We never really know until the actual colon is biopsied. It's kind of the ultimate biopsy."

I am left with a lingering doubt as to whether this is actually going to be over. If the biopsy reveals Crohn's disease, it means the surgery was not curative, and there is no known cure. Again, I am in that emotional state where I'm too wound up and overwhelmed to feel anything. So I go into academic mode and quiz him for details. He respectfully answers every single question. He sits with me for about twenty minutes, which is a lifetime in hospital-land. I admit to him that I don't really care about having the catheter removed because I'm still maintaining full bladder control and I want to move around anyway. He laughs but maintains the nurse's stand that it must have been put in wrong. I forgive him for the discussion about "the" colon, though I don't tell him that I remember.

He asks me when I'm going to get the second surgery done to remove the rest of my sigmoid colon and my rectum and reverse the ileostomy. Healthier, less steroid-dependent patients can have the entire surgery done as one procedure. I have already decided to pretend that I had that surgery to avoid the "bag-lady" look—which is how I presume everyone looks at you when you've had your colon removed.

I tell him that I'm not sure, but my understanding is that there is no rush.

"Well, no, you don't have to do it right away...but sooner is better than later because of your cancer risk."

"Um, yes, my cancer risk."

I know it's higher than the average person, both because of the severity of my colitis and because people on both sides of my family have died of colon cancer. But I didn't think the risk was an immediate concern before this. I hold this new information tightly in my chest, afraid that, if I let it sink into the depths of my emotional being, I will completely dissolve. So I remain stoic, calm, and competent.

When Athena, the surgeon, comes to visit me, she's pleased that I have given back the morphine pump and that I'm just taking the occasional Tylenol for pain. She proudly tells her accompanying resident that this is the advantage of being able to perform the surgery laparoscopically. She puts me on a clear liquids diet and says that, if it goes well, I can go onto solid food in the morning.

13. Without Hope

The final morning. Final rounds. My final chance to impart my patient insights to the medical students gathered around my bed.

"Could you please wait a minute? I have something to say."

"Sure!" said the Cheshire Cat Resident with his standard grin.

"I don't want to be pedantic, but I'd like to make a point about pain tolerance in colitis patients."

Blank, irritated stares.

"It seemed to me that, whenever I was admitted to the hospital, nobody really acknowledged how much pain I was in. Then, I would go into scopes, where the medication never worked, and they told me, 'This shouldn't be causing you so much pain.' But it did. And now, when I come out of surgery, everyone is shocked that I stopped pushing the morphine button. Because Tylenol is fine. This isn't really that painful comparatively. Colitis patients withstand a great deal of pain."

When I stop for a breath, they all start briskly walking out. Cat boy says, "Good to know! More Fentenil for my scope patients!"

Until this moment, I'm using all of my strength to keep myself in a somewhat upright sitting position. As they leave, I flop backwards onto the mattress and cover my face with my hands. I'm embarrassed that I have exposed myself to what feels like their ridicule and shaming. I'm enraged that my observations from *inside* the body they're gazing down at are being completely ignored. I'm fading away into a bleak, hopeless, grey space — moving through swirling shapes and shadows in what feels like endless empty space.

"Jules!"

I snap back to the hospital bed. "What?"

Frida is sitting next to me, her arm loosely draped across my hips. She puts her other hand on my cheek. "Come back to earth!"

"I don't want to!"

"I'm going to tell you something very important. Right now." She leans in. "You have work to do." Her tone is gentle, but there's a forceful insistence behind her words.

"Work to do?" I ask. "I have nothing to do. No voice. Nothing to say. No one cares."

"Do you think you're the only person to feel this way?" She asks. "I heard what that resident said to you this morning. Do you really think you have nothing to teach them?"

I think back, remembering the moment she must be referring to. They arrived at my bed while I was using the washroom. When I walked out, with no hook-ups, dressed in my own pyjamas and slippers, Cheshire Cat Resident said, "Look at you, you're human again!"

At the time, I dismissed it, thinking, he's probably met many patients who described the grimy, restricted feeling of being in hospital as "inhuman."

Frida is looking into my eyes at this point, watching the scene as it flits across my memory. She demands, "So what do you think about that now?"

"I think he betrays his general, if not entirely conscious, mental distinction between The Sick and The Healthy. I am now the Subtotal Colectomy. Less than total. Not quite human. Incomplete." The words come out of my mouth as if they've been thought by someone else, in some other place.

"Write it down," she tells me. "Write it down."

In this moment, I develop my new life ambition: to lecture masses of med students, to teach future clinicians—possibly always wearing a hospital gown. I want to give voice to the sheeted slab on the operating table, the gowned exhibit in the bed.

14. Reformed

So I go home, with my subtotal colectomy and end-ileostomy. Less and more, reformed, re-formed. The nervous system that regulates the GI tract is supposed to be comparable to a brain — am I now partly lobotomized? I am concerned that my lack of guts will inhibit my capacity to have "gut" feelings. But the phantom colon quickly resurrects itself. As the visceral feelings of anxiety and fear return to my abdomen, I wonder why I would ever resent their loss.

All the concepts associated with my intestines are flooding into my mind as I try desperately to rationalize my new form. Having guts...having no guts...or less guts...gutting fish. Having my guts exposed. Being gutted.

To the surprising number of people who've told me, "Man, you've got balls," I've always responded, "No, no, I've got fallopian tubes. It seems they're working quite well." But I never minded musings on my "gutsy" bravery. So now, has the mouthy, gutsy woman been reformed?

When I was in high school, I had a friend whose brother was taking visual art in university. He would bring home film student productions, and we would go over and watch them. One of them involved a man who was very, very bored. He walked around his apartment, and after being incapable of finding any satisfying entertainment, he took out a knife and literally disembowelled himself. He first cut a small hole, then the rest of the film entailed him slowly pulling out his intestines, forming a giant pile in front of him. When I imagine my ileostomy under my clothes, this film image is all I see. A surgeon cut a hole in my stomach, pulled my intestines out, and left me in a state of disbelief and bewilderment, caring for the dangling remnant poking through.

After my warm and fuzzy experience in the hospital with the nurses and the Bag, I decide not to consent to home care. But a nurse named Dinah phones an hour after I get home from the hospital to tell me that she's coming at noon the next day. The next morning, I decide to phone and cancel, but the doorbell rings at 10:30 a.m., and there she is. She bustles in with confidence and authority, and is so at ease that her demeanour is contagious. It turns out she's funny, lewd, and crude, everything a good nurse should be.

She asks what I've named my stoma and we debate possibilities for some time. I tell her about being able to control my catheter. It turns out that she has similar talents. With her, though, they were so insistent that it must have been put in wrong that they took it out and put it in again. When she could still control it, they finally conceded that she must have some special muscular powers in her bladder.

She gives me piles and piles of literature, Kegel exercises to keep my sphincter muscle working to get ready for the next operation, and tips on everything I need to look out for while caring for my stoma. The literature refers to patients with stomas as "Ostomates." I am appalled by the title and Dinah is sympathetic.

"I hate that word...I can't believe they still use it." Clearly in tune with her patients, Dinah is offended for all of us at such a dehumanizing label.

The device I brought home from the hospital is a "two piece." The top piece of plastic is pasted around the stoma, and the bag is attached with a Tupperware-like seal. A clip at the bottom allows drainage, and the entire bag can be removed for cleaning the stoma between the twice-weekly changes.

But I can't look at it without gagging. It's inflamed and mangled. After taking one look at my face while cleaning it, Dinah says, "Okay, it's okay. I'll do it this time…"

The thing that grosses me out the most is the process of measuring the stoma. Because it's still healing, it's supposed to get smaller every time we change the bag. So, on the back of the bag, there are varying sizes of circles to cut out an opening that fits snugly around the stoma.

Dinah teaches me to measure by putting a thin piece of cardboard with pre-cut circles around the stoma to see which one fits. The feeling of thin cardboard scraping against my stoma sends shivers through my body. I have physical memories of the paper cuts that perpetually plagued my hands when I worked at a card store in high school. Except this time, the paper cuts aren't going to be on my fingers.

I explain to Dinah, "I just had no idea what it was going to look like. Maybe I should have looked at the pictures everyone kept trying to show me in the pre-op appointment. I was picturing the tracheotomy in the disembodied neck being used as a cautionary tale in the anti-smoking commercial, not a bright red dangling piece of intestine that bleeds every time you touch it and sputters liquid shit!"

She's sympathetic. "I know, it's a big adjustment. I'll do it for today. I promise, it gets easier. There are layers and layers of blood vessels right at the surface, so the bleeding is normal. It's nothing to worry about."

It would take some serious mental acrobatics for me to ever accept any of this as normal. I'd say it's highly unusual to have to wipe the blood off my stomach that's actually dripping from my protruding small intestine. It occurs to me that the nurses and doctors are doing what psychiatrists refer to as "self-reporting." Like when someone says, "I wasn't scared," even though no one asked them if they were. They wouldn't have even brought it up if they weren't. The perpetual obsession with denying my abnormality simply highlights it in my mind.

The plastic seal between my stomach and the adhesively attached "appliance" is supposed to be air- and watertight. But twice I wake up in the night to a horrific smell, to find leaks all over my abdomen. I figure I must have done something to it in my sleep, and I don't want to leave the house in case this happens in the outside world.

15. Big Mouth

One evening, while I'm still feeling very insecure about all of this, my parents' friends come to visit. Apparently they are here to see me, but I'm really not feeling up to seeing anyone. My dad insists that I'm being rude, staying upstairs and watching TV with Blair when I should be socializing with guests, so I reluctantly concede and go entertain my well-wishers. I wonder how often this happens when people aren't well: having to socialize when we'd rather be left alone. There's so much tradition and protocol around visiting people in hospitals and after surgery. But for me, I think a lot of that is about allaying the anxiety of healthy visitors who want to see for themselves how *we*'re doing. The idea that it's "rude" to set boundaries and take a stance about what kind of socializing is appropriate really prevents us from taking care of ourselves when we're ill.

Ultimately, I find that I can't maintain my "taking it badly" stand for very long. It is hard work sulking about visitors and complaining to the nurses about how gross the whole ileostomy thing is. It really is more work than stoically taking it well. So I decide to become an expert at cleaning and changing the stoma and bag. I also demand smaller sized one-piece bags with no potential for leakage because they are pasted directly to the skin. Dinah is very impressed with my quick turnaround.

She tells the nurse she brought with her, "Last time I thought she was going to retch!"

To me, she says admiringly, "I know you think it's really gross, but you do have a nice stoma."

Dinah is deeply biased in favour of female surgeons. "I don't know what it is, the attention to detail, she just makes them point exactly the right way. The male surgeons don't care; they don't even think about it. It makes such a huge difference in quality of life for patients."

This is when I finally admit, quietly, because I'm sure she's going to think I'm crazy, that I can feel the stoma. I have read and been told repeatedly that I'm not supposed to be able to feel it. The only thing that we Ostomates are supposed to feel is the skin around it. I considered this possibility at some length, but the difference between the feeling of something touching external skin on my tummy and the feeling of something touching my intestine is unmistakable.

Dinah, who thus far has taken everything in her stride, looks at me like I've cracked.

"Really? But there's no nerves there…"

"Yes," I say defiantly. "If you want, I'll look away while you clean it. I'll tell you when you're touching it and when you're not."

It's the first time I've taken my infamous "tone" with her.

"It's okay," she says. "I believe you. It's just that I've never heard of that; it's very rare. You must have a hypersensitive bowel. You really shouldn't be able to feel it."

I breathe a sigh of relief. Dinah had not in fact turned into Automaton Nurse who denies any difference in patient experience. On our final visit, she has a student nurse with her.

Dinah encourages me. "Tell her what you said to the med students!"

So I repeat the story and they both laugh with glee — and in horror — about the Cheshire Cat Resident.

"You really need to write this down," Dinah tells me. "And I want to be in the book. Write me in, okay?"

"Don't worry." I assure her. "It's all going in and you'll be a star."

In the meantime, my friends are convincing me that no one can see anything through my clothes and that they aren't even thinking about my stoma, that it's safe to go out. The first day that I wear fitted pants with a fitted sweater I am at a party. I walk into the kitchen to look and see if there's anything cooking I can eat. I'm still on a no-insoluble-fibre diet because the post-surgical inflammation in my bowel can cause blockages if I eat anything that's difficult to digest. Innocently looking in the pots, I ask the guy stirring one of them what the ingredients are. It's all vegetarian food, high on fibre, low on safe digestion.

He says, "Oh, that's right, your diet is restricted. You know, John's brother had the same thing as you."

"Yes, I know."

I'm really not up for this conversation and am trying to be as short as possible, hoping he gets the point.

He launches into quizzing me about my water retention from the steroids.

"Yep, John's brother got really bloated."

"Mmm," I say. "But it all goes away when you come off of them."

I picture the conversation where people wondered if I was on the same medication as John's brother, discussing the "cushnoid face" and "obese abdomen" that Dr. Bird faithfully recorded in my medical chart.

And then, when I think it can't get any worse, he slaps his own abdomen in the exact spot my stoma is located on me and loudly, with a booming voice, in a crowded kitchen, asks, "*So*, how long are you going to be on the bag then?"

Suddenly, the kitchen explodes into a tornado, sucking all the air from my lungs and strength from my limbs. I try to muster the best school teacher look I can, frozen in shock, one eyebrow slightly raised, hoping he will realize the gravity of the horrific thing he has just asked. He looks back blankly, still waiting for a response.

"I don't have a bag," I say squarely.

"Oh, really" he says, "because..."

He's clearly ready to argue with me, and I'm not sure if he's planning to interrogate me until I admit it, but I cut him off before he has a chance. "They do it all internally these days."

I wander off, somewhat aimlessly, not sure what to do, wanting to leave.

Estelle, my friend who dubbed me Bionic Woman a few months earlier, wants to see the backyard, so I go with her. I tell her what the guy said and that I just want to go home. To escape through the back gate because surely he knows. And everybody knows. And even though I can't see it, there's a bulging bag of shit stretching the material on my pants. And that's all anyone can see or think when they look at me. Ostomate.

And she says, "No. You're not leaving. No one knows. He's appalling, ridiculous. You're not getting pushed out of here by him." She says that, even though she knew it was there, it hadn't even occurred to her. "You don't look like someone who had surgery. You just seem so confident; no one would guess."

She wants to go talk to him, but seeing as I made such a point of saying I didn't have a bag, it seemed a bit self-defeating to have someone go and tell him how inappropriate it was to ask about my (non-)bag. So this is what my life has become, leaving parties to cry in people's backyards. I didn't even do this in high school. It's like the revenge of the teenage hormones that I managed to resist until I was twenty-four.

We make our way around the house to the front of the porch, where Estelle's husband is smoking. I tell him the story and he unleashes a long line of expletives. He tells me a story about a guy he once knew smashing another guy's head through a microwave door for saying something gross about a female friend who'd had the same surgery as me. And even though I know Estelle's husband isn't offering to smash Big Mouth's giant head through glass, the macho image appeals to me. I laugh, feel better, and re-join the party.

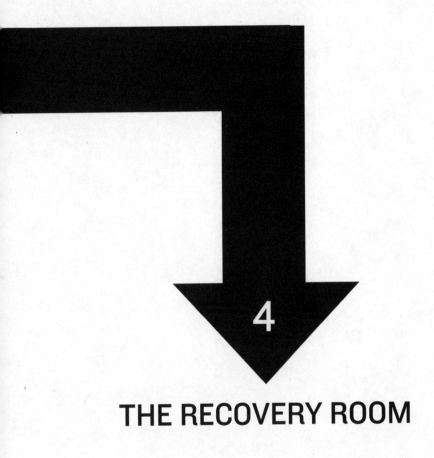

4

THE RECOVERY ROOM

I. Back to Oz

Frances learns something in this moment that will allow
her to survive and function for the rest of her life. She finds
out that one thing can look like another. That the facts of a
situation don't necessarily indicate anything about the truth
of the situation. In this moment, fact and truth become
separated and commence to wander like twins in a fairy-
tale, waiting to be reunited by that special someone who
possesses the secret of telling them apart.
— Ann-Marie MacDonald, *Fall on Your Knees*

Three weeks after my operation, in the middle of what is expected to be a
six-week recovery, I fly back to Vancouver. Before the surgery, I had decided
that I wanted to finish my master's degree. Tara still wants to supervise me
and feels that the courses I took in Toronto are totally applicable to what
I'm studying. Another professor I really like is teaching the only mandatory
course I have left to do, and my friend Ethan, who's still in med school
in Vancouver, has recommended another really interesting professor for
my last elective course. I've contacted both profs and they're both more
than happy to have me in their classes. It seems so straightforward. I'll

arrive in January and take three courses with three agreeable professors, then come back to Toronto in April to write my thesis.

When I get home after my surgery, I discover that my department disagrees. They want me to apply all over again with all the other applicants for the following academic year. That means September. They explain that this process is "just to be fair to everyone."

One night, Maia comes over. "I just feel so helpless from here," I tell her. "I wish I could just go in person and meet with these people."

She offers to book a flight for me to Vancouver so I can sort this mess out in person. She's so generous like this. We book the ticket, and I fly out the next morning. It's hard. I don't really sleep much from the time we book the flight until I get back to Toronto six days later. The steroid withdrawal gives me moments of nausea and dizziness, and I begin my first flare-up of rectal disease. Urgent, bloody, painful discharge. I thought once my colon was removed, everything would settle down. But despite the fact that no food is passing through this small stump of leftover rectum, my immune system has decided it is a threat. So the internal attack continues.

I land in Vancouver with a rage so tangible it makes my arms numb. With all the build-up about going back, it is strange to feel as if I've never left. I've forgotten about the startling vacuity of the beauty. The mountains and ocean seem to taunt me, when the rest of my life is so disappointingly removed from the scenery all around me. The sterility is suffocating. I remember the craving I felt during the winter I spent in Vancouver—to walk in the gritty, slushy Toronto snow sloshing between the streetcar tracks. Vancouver has no smell.

The sun is shining, but the wind is cold. I go straight from the airport to the university and meet Ethan. He wants me to carry my colon around in a jar. Emphatically slamming it down on counters and desktops when anyone gives me a hard time. It's a joke Blair makes whenever anything stresses me out. "Uh-oh, Julie's colon is twitching in its jar somewhere." We go to the student union office and meet one of the vice-presidents,

Jonny. I know him from the occupation of the president's office a year and a half earlier. Jonny and I walk over to the dean's office. It's super-fancy and intimidating. I look around, not even sure where I'd begin to address anyone here. Jonny heads straight over to the phone in the lobby and picks it up, Michael Moore style, dialling the dean's direct extension.

"Gretchen? Jon Mansfield here, VP administration for the student union. I've got Julie Devaney here from Toronto. We would like to follow up on the letter she wrote three weeks ago."

She agrees to meet with us. I notice that I'm shaking as we walk to her office. We sit in front of her and I mentally coach myself, *Be nice, be nice, deferential, sympathetic.*

She says that the Dean's Office would certainly support my readmission for January but that they need a recommendation from the department. She informs me that I wouldn't actually want "reinstatement" because I would have to pay back fees for the time I missed, so to let my department know that I actually want a "friendly readmission" with a retroactive medical leave for the time I missed.

We walk over to the women's studies department. The ghost of Julie, slightly less visible, slightly less real, ready to elicit the horror and fear that apparitions tend to do. Back to haunt them.

Snot-Face is still the director of the department. When I approach her in the hallway, she looks right through me. "Can I help you?"

I play along without even a hint of sarcasm colouring my tone. "Oh, I guess you don't remember me." I smile brightly and stretch my hand toward her. "Julie Devaney. I was enrolled in the MA here a year and a half ago, and I'm interested in coming back in January."

I am perfectly aware that she knows exactly who I am and why I'm there.

"Yes," she replies coldly. "I know who you are. Do you have an appointment?"

I explain that I've just arrived from Toronto and met with the Dean's Office.

"Well, you'll have to speak to the graduate advisor, and she's away. That's why it's always important to make appointments," she replies darkly.

The department secretary takes my cellphone number and agrees to try and get in touch with the graduate advisor. She promises that she'll let me know if she hears anything and that she'll try to get me an appointment for Friday. It's Wednesday.

The next morning, I wake up in pain, nauseated, and with no output in my bag. This has never happened before. My abdomen is bloated and harder than usual. It's almost certainly a bowel blockage. I lie down, massaging my belly, plying myself with warm mint tea. Finally, hours later, there is movement in the bag. It oozes out thick and dry like cottage cheese. The blockage has passed without me having to wade into the horror of Vancouver emergency rooms—without me having to endure the humiliation of admitting that I have been rash and foolish to travel across the country in my weakened state, or the guilt of having to worry everyone after so firmly asserting that I'm "fine."

I have a good day wandering around Susie's favourite beach playing with people's dogs. Whenever the pain gets too intense, I retreat into coffee shops and drink more mint tea. I find comfortable pieces of driftwood to sit on while I settle into my novel. As the waves wash up on the shore, I remember the dreams I had under anaesthetic. The place I was sitting was at the base of the street we had lived on in Vancouver. The shoreline from there went directly to the university. In my dream, I was walking west, toward the school, involuntarily holding my breath. Now as write this, I can't remember which sensations and thoughts were in that moment and which I only dreamed. The smell of the beach, the sound and feelings of the moving air and waves, and the overwhelming sense that I had forgotten something important, something that I used to know.

A young woman and her dog are walking between the water's edge and me. The dog has the physical characteristics of a stereotypical attack dog, but I can tell by its manner that it's friendly. I call out and the dog comes bounding. The woman follows and immediately notes what I'm reading.

"*Fall on Your Knees!*" she exclaims. "I loved that book."

Both my friend Martine and my Aunt Mary gave me copies to read while I was recovering from my surgery. I agree with her, and she thanks me for playing with her dog and moves on.

Every time I feel a draft or movement of cold, which is often in damp Vancouver, my legs cramp up. Soon my rectum starts spasming and pains shoot up into my tailbone. If I am indoors, I can try and cover my legs with my fake fur-lined coat. This helps a bit. Sitting on a heating pad is best. If I am outside, I just cramp and shiver, shiver and cramp. I can't tell which is causing the other.

Friday is supposed to be the day of truth. I phone the department when I wake up. The friendly secretary from two days earlier is now openly hostile. I can't help wondering who told her that I eat kittens.

"I have your cellphone number. If I know anything, I'll call you. There's no need to come in again. If we can't arrange a meeting with anyone before you leave, you'll just have to continue this discussion over email."

It's trial by rumour. I invaded their playground and they're certainly not going to let me get my hands on the ball.

I have a good weekend with my friends, and then Monday rolls in. I meet up with Jonny, who's insistent that we go into the department, whether or not they've called me back. It's pouring rain, but luckily Jonny's umbrella is big enough to share.

The secretary looks scared, like we might have just gotten her into a lot of trouble. It seems to be her job to put off the pesky ex-student who keeps hassling everyone about discrimination. She has decisively failed. She tells us that she'll phone the graduate advisor, whose office is in another building, and let us know if she's available.

"Don't bother," Jonny says. "We'll just go over there if that's where she is."

The secretary looks at us sternly as if we're a pair of recalcitrant five-year-olds. "No, wait there." She points at a bench in the entranceway.

Forget about being a kitten-eater—I'm starting to think that someone told her that I'm a serial killer. This is where the irony of the reference strikes me. One of Blair's favourite shows is the HBO series *Oz*, about Oswald state prison. Blair will often try to woo me into watching it with promises of astute and incisive illustrations of the prison-industrial complex. I agree, the politics are great, but the content is too traumatic. So now, the magical promise of my deepest educational desire has turned into imprisonment. *Oz* meets Oswald in the department lobby.

While we wait, Mitzi walks in, the colour draining from her face at the sight of me. *A spectre is haunting the university—the spectre of a rude little activist. All the powers of the old Academy have entered into a holy alliance to exorcise it...*

I smile brightly. "Hi!"

She gives a shaky half-smile back, mumbling a "Hello" as she rushes off.

My mind travels back to the first clue I got that I don't belong here. The very first time I entered this building in September 2001—when the director of the department sat us down and told of the reams of applications they had received for our spots, the seven little MA students worthy of their program. The message was clear. Yes, be proud of yourselves, but be grateful, because plenty of others would take your place. I don't know what *their* first clue was that I didn't belong here—probably somewhere between organizing a sit-in and refusing to accept their unjust decrees.

As we wait and wait on the bench, Jonny becomes increasingly impatient. I'm now accustomed to being treated this way, but Jonny is outraged.

"You're here from Toronto. You just had major surgery and you just want to talk to them. We're just going over there, to her office, now."

So we get up, say goodbye to the secretary, and head over to the graduate advisor's office. When we arrive, her office is locked. Her colleague in the next office comes out, puzzled.

"She was just here; this is her office hour. Her coat's there, her computer's on—I don't know where she could be."

She fled the scene with the warning that we were coming.

With memories of the occupation of the president's office dancing in our heads, we sit down on the cold hallway tile. And wait.

Forty-five minutes later, the woman of the vanishing office hour comes rushing back. She looks through me and the student union rep at another waiting student and smiles.

"Come on in."

"Oh, no, they were here first, and if you don't have time, I'll just email you. It's okay."

So the graduate advisor is stuck. Forced to deal with this matter that she's been so steadfastly avoiding for so long.

Top Ten Rules to Being a Good Bureaucrat:

10) When escaping, take your car keys.

9) Turn off your computer monitor, or at least close your inbox.

Well, that's two, anyway. I don't actually know how to be a good bureaucrat. I just know that she is failing miserably. The first thing Jonny notices is the repeated emails in her inbox with the subject line "Julie Devaney" that have been opened and replied to.

I'm in too much of a panic to notice anything so useful. I can't even describe the office, and I wouldn't recognize her if I met her again. I just remember shapes and shadows. I'm friendly, meek, apologetic. I can see exactly what is going through her mind, nakedly exposed in the worry lines on her face...*I'm an academic. I write books, teach courses. I took this bureaucratic post that I don't have time for. It was supposed to be easy. I don't want to deal with this. No no no no no no.* If she could close her eyes, tap her heels together, and send me back to Toronto, she would.

"But I don't know you," she says when I say that surely there should be no issue in re-admitting me.

This is apparently a legitimate factor to her. She doesn't need to *know*

me. It's within the realm of human rights legislation that with the information I've provided, they have to accommodate me. She knows my
academic standing, my program of study, and the support I have from the
faculty members I want to work with.

She even admits, "Well, Tara was very positive about you when I asked."

I'm just so confounded. I don't understand the rules to this game.
What else does she need to know? It's not supposed to be a matter of
her personal judgment whether I should be allowed to finish my degree.

Then she starts to interrogate me. As if, by asking me the same question
enough different ways, I'll suddenly reveal that I've been lying all along.
I finally break down after being asked to repeat for the tenth time why I
left a year earlier. But tears have no effect on her. I later tell Ethan that
the most tragic casualty of this incident is my pretty gold eyeshadow, which
is now unattractively smeared over my cheeks. She waits at least a minute
and a half before impatiently offering me a tissue.

"Here."

At this point, she starts quizzing me about my academic plans and field
of study. My complete breakdown has no effect on my ability to articulate
my research interests. A generally unhealthy detachment between intellect
and emotions is finally proving useful. But I'm angry, humiliated, disgusted.
I can't understand what anyone could possibly have said about me that
would give her the confidence to so vilely trample the boundaries of
respect. There's a twenty-four-year-old woman sitting in front of her crying
after spending the last year and a half in and out of hospitals, getting cut
up. And she's coldly quizzing me about my thesis topic.

Finally, she interrupts me, looking at her watch.

"I have to go and pick my son up from school. Poor little guy. We don't
want him waiting in the rain."

She makes a cutesy, scrunched-up face at me like I'm supposed to
express some kind of sympathy for her *poor little guy*.

When I don't, she abruptly stands up. "We'll certainly look at this issue again," she says. "We'll let you know."

She tries to hand back the letter of support I gave her from the Disability Resource Centre.

"No, that's yours." I say and hand it back to her, puzzled.

She'd looked at the letter when I first gave it to her; she must have seen that it's addressed to her personally, but she's so absorbed by the impulse to not deal with it, to make me go away, that she's not acting reasonably.

I fly back to Toronto the next day. I get into a bit of trouble from Dinah, my home care nurse, when I see her. First, she's pleased that I've gone to fight and has to be restrained from getting on a plane to go and take them down herself. But she's less enthusiastic when examining the swelling around my stoma site. "What have you been doing? Have you been working out? Have you been lifting heavy things? This kind of localized inflammation really isn't good. It could mean there's a lot more internal inflammation."

But as I rest over the next few days, the inflammation does subside.

In the following weeks, I get a letter from Snot-Face, stating that if I want to come back, I have to pay all the tuition from the time I was gone. It's thousands and thousands of dollars I don't have for time that I was sick and hospitalized. The letter includes her threateningly telling me that I'll have to do all the same coursework and readings as everyone else. As if I'm somehow unaware that graduate work entails reading. The obvious implication throughout being, "We know you're trying to get one over on us."

I phone my advisor at the Disability Resource Centre and tell her about the letter. Her response is, "Well, that's punitive."

I phone the dean directly on her extension. I outline the situation and explain why it's clearly discriminatory. I say that I realize it must seem strange that I am contacting her when it seems that it would be more appropriate to talk to my department, but that they are not being very helpful or straightforward with me. She agrees that it's punitive and promises to look into getting me a retroactive medical leave.

The politics of institutional re-admittance in universities and hospitals are almost identical: confession and penance. Medical doctors, Doctors of Philosophy. Their approach to my illness has a great deal in common with the Catholic approach to a sinner. Bare your soul, disclose the intimate details of your disease, and we'll consider helping you. But, first, you will be punished. And then you will be forever indebted to us for achieving our forgiveness.

Bless me, Doctor, for I have sinned. It has been many months since I was a productive economic unit. Please forgive me the following trespasses . . .

2. System Failure

A few weeks later, I go to see Athena, the surgeon, for my follow-up appointment. I imagine wild and ridiculous things as I walk down the hall to her office. No one called me with the results from the pathology report when they biopsied my colon. Deep within me is a cringing little child, terrified that the report came back saying nothing is wrong with me and (difficult as this part is to admit) that there would be law enforcement officers waiting to charge me with massive defrauding of the health care system. There's definitely an element of fanciful drama, but at the same time, I'm not thinking these thoughts; they're thinking me.

I ask Dawn later, very quietly, on the phone, "Can I tell you what I was thinking when I was going to my surgeon's appointment?"

"Sure," she says.

So I tell her. Shockingly, she starts to cry. "Look at what these bastards have done to you. Do you realize what they've done to you? They've convinced you. You've internalized all their crap."

As she cries, I think back throughout my long illness. Anytime anything made me happy, I would feel guilty. If I was enjoying any attention, appreciating the quiet that gave me time to read, space to think that I had never had in my über-busy health, I was convinced that I was putting everyone through the stress and worry of my illness while I was secretly getting something out of it. And if I liked it, then surely I had done this to myself. Of course, it sounds absurd written down like this, but as a deep belief that's impossible to shake, it's profound and concrete. And the guilt is regularly reinforced by people with institutional power addressing me with an air of blame, as if I had done something shameful and bad.

Of course, the pathology report comes back to say that I had ulcerative colitis.

"So that's good," my surgeon says casually.

I know what she means; it's good that the diagnosis was correct. If I actually had Crohn's disease, it would mean that my entire GI tract, from mouth to anus, at every level (not just the mucosa), would be affected by the disease. Such a scenario would render my "curative" surgery quite useless in the ultimate progress of my illness. But "good" still isn't exactly the word I would pick to describe the confirmation.

Athena agrees that I can go back to Vancouver to finish my program. She warns that after being on such high doses of steroids for so long, I may need to go back onto five milligrams for a while. She doesn't really explain anymore. She just says, "Well, it's a good sign that you're feeling okay now, but if you find you're peeing all the time and you can't get out of bed in the morning, it means you need to go back on five milligrams."

I tell her that I need a letter outlining my disease, surgery, and prognosis for the university, and I have a suggested draft written. She looks over my printed copy and says, "This is great. Just email it to us and we'll print it on our letterhead and send it in."

Then I tell her what Dinah said about how much she loves her stoma-construction talents. Athena laughs.

"Dinah says women surgeons do a better job," I tell her.

She modestly rolls her eyes, "I don't think it's a matter of gender..."

I just shrug. But I think Dinah, the stoma-nurse, may have point—she's obviously got a huge sample from which to judge.

When I get home that night, there's an email from the graduate advisor at the university. She says the only way they'll process my request is if I produce *medical documents* stating that I was advised to withdraw instead of take a medical leave. Nobody in Vancouver had treated me. That's why I needed to leave when I did. My family doctor had closed his practice; my specialist passed me on to another specialist, who passed me on to a surgeon. Who's going to produce this letter?

I can't sleep at all that night. At five in the morning, I sit down and write the letters—one with all the explicit medical details that the Disability Resource Centre wants so they can justify my legitimacy as an "authentic" sick person, and one with all the timelines, stating that I was advised to move back to Toronto.

The woman who runs my surgeon's office is a goddess. When I phone to see if she was able to open the attachments, she shares her outrage with me.

"You shouldn't have to deal with these people!" she says.

She prints the letters word for word on the letterhead from Athena's office. She adds a line at the end that if the university has any questions whatsoever, they should feel free to phone Athena directly. She catches Athena between operations and has her sign them. She faxes them directly to the university and even follows up on the phone to make sure they've received them. I'm so incredibly thankful.

And it occurs to me that I shouldn't have to be so grateful that one institution has provided accurate and truthful information to another institution about me. But I am. If I had known the fight with the university would involve, and how much effort it would take, I never would have taken it on. I was just thinking that every step would be the last. And finally it is. Nobody gets in touch with me to tell me that I've won. I simply check the student service website, and when I enter my student number, I find that my registration has been reactivated, and when I try to enrol in my courses, I am successful. I email the dean's office, and they confirm that this is the case.

I've been completely off the steroids for a few weeks. I'm feeling increasingly tired, depressed, out of sorts, and I'm having trouble remembering things. I start reading medical encyclopedias that outline the conditions for adrenal failure. I'm frustrated that no one described this process to me in any useful detail. Adrenal glands can atrophy and shrink from extended use of high-dose steroid treatment. No one ever told me that part. How do you grow a gland back? Apparently, when your adrenal glands stop producing cortisol, your body doesn't register this until you are 90 percent depleted. It happens so gradually that, at first, you just think you're a bit tired, a bit dizzy, a bit nauseated. Maybe you have some muscle pain, abdominal pain. But usually, people don't realize until they are in some kind of major crisis, and the body can't cope because the resource we use to deal with stress, our cortisol, has very slowly disappeared. And then you die.

When all of these symptoms gradually come on, I first put them down to potassium and sodium depletion from my missing colon. I eat more potassium-rich and high-sodium foods. Then I get my period, so I assume that's why I'm feeling crappy. It's Christmas day when I finally admit to myself that my body is shutting down. I need to nap in the afternoon. When it's time for dinner, my mum calls me down, but I can't move. Every cell rages with pain. When I finally stand up, I feel like I may collapse, so I go back to bed. I know then that I'm going to have to go back onto the steroids. As I lie there exhausted, I burst into tears. I cry and cry and cry because I'm so done with this. So finished with being ill. So completely done with coping.

I dutifully go back on five milligrams of steroids and immediately start to feel better. Within days, I am approaching "normal" again. I go to see the doctor who has taken over my family doctor's practice. He's sure that if I stay on that dose for the four months I'm in Vancouver, I'll be fine. I want to be sure, so I question him.

"But every time I stabilized on one dose before it would at some point stop working. What if that happens again?"

He gives me The Look that I've become oh-so familiar with from health care professionals. "That was your colitis; this is completely different."

I drop the issue. I want him to be right anyway.

Getting ready to go to Vancouver, I can't pack. The morning I'm leaving, I sit in the hallway with piles and piles of clothes and papers and books and no idea what to do with any of it. Maia and Blair end up packing for me. Blair takes me to the airport.

A strange thing occurs on the plane. I'm chatting animatedly with my seatmate who I stupidly assume is gay, based on his mannerisms and his size-small hooded sweatshirt. It's not because men who are his actual physical size tend to be gay; it's more because, in 2003, straight men don't tend to *admit* to being a size small, and would buy the medium. I guess he's a hipster before his time. It turns out he's on his way to a faraway land to enthusiastically join the army. It also turns out that he's going to be in Vancouver for a few days and is looking for some female companionship. But that really isn't the point. The point is that he says to me, "You should never plan anything. When you plan things they never work out like you think they will, and then you're disappointed."

I privately think this is a very ill-conceived notion. After all, I plan everything, and look at how well things are going, despite all the obstacles put in my way. But I don't say this. I just pretend to be very interested in the movie to get out of the fact that he is quite directly trying to make plans with me for that evening. But as it turns out, he's my Sibyl. Prophets and soothsayers always come in the most unlikely of shells. It's strangely appropriate that mine is a soldier in a size-small hoodie.

When I arrive in Vancouver, I immediately have a headache. Adrian and Ethan come and pick me up from the airport and we go out for dinner. I start feeling really nauseated. But the sicker I feel, the more muddled my brain is. Confused thoughts colliding. When I go up to my loft, I unpack my sleeping bag and blanket, some warm sweat pants and a sweater. I try really hard to ignore the fact that the entire apartment is spinning. I don't want to acknowledge the extreme nausea that is washing through my body. Or the pounding of my head and my leaden muscles and aching joints.

Then I discover that the plumbing isn't working. Without getting into the disgusting details, and please, let me assure you this is way grosser to experience than to read, I now have diarrhea filling up my ileostomy bag. I phone the other tenant to tell her that my plumbing isn't working. "Oh, it is really cold," she says. "Your pipes must have frozen. Let me bring you some tea."

So she brings me mint tea and some containers filled with water. When she leaves, I take some Gravol and sip steadfastly on the tea. I try to fall asleep in the bed, but it is way too cold. I push the little couch next to the tiny base heater that is on full blast and heating the area about three inches in front of it with astounding efficiency. I spend the rest of the night on the little couch, fading in and out of consciousness, extremely confused, alternately vomiting and shivering violently. With a toilet that doesn't flush. I think the freezing cold is probably the only thing that brings me to.

Around 6:30 in the morning, I phone my mum, who's at work in Toronto, where it's 9:30 a.m.

"You have to get out of there."

"I'm coming home."

"People always feel like that when they start something new. Don't be impulsive, you've worked so hard to get back there. Do you have somewhere to go in Vancouver?"

But it's not just a matter of being scared and out of sorts. My body knows. This is shutdown mode, and it's not going away. Blacking out isn't normal. Blacking out in the middle of the night while living alone is scary. I don't tell my mum or anyone else how seriously ill I am and certainly not that I've been losing consciousness. I am more terrified of ending up stranded in a Vancouver hospital than I am about anything happening in my body.

I can't remember much of anything that happened; I don't really know how I got onto the plane. I remember taking a cab to my friend Adrian's apartment after I got off the phone with my mum. I slept a lot. Adrian borrowed a car and helped me pick my things up from the loft. I returned my keys to the other tenant, booked a flight on the Internet, and was gone within thirty-six hours of arriving. I was completely on autopilot. I just knew I needed to go home.

3. Home...Again

My plane lands in Toronto.

Blair is waiting at the airport in his new puffy black jacket. I last saw him fifty-six hours earlier, but it feels like years. I wish that books had soundtracks so I could play Aimee Mann's live cover of "The Scientist" and have a subtly constructed soppy airport scene.

But you'll just have to imagine it.

We get home, and Willow Rosenberg, the kitten, does back flips and somersaults. Apparently she's been lying on the bench by the front door, staring mournfully at the handle the whole time I've been gone. She has carried a giant, rolled-up pair of woollen socks down the stairs, socks that I wore before I left. They are literally more than half the size of her little kitten body.

My family doctor gets me an appointment to see an endocrinologist, the type of doctor who deals with hormones and adrenal glands. I've independently upped the dose of my steroids, so I trust that I'll be okay until someone figures out a tapering schedule that won't kill me. I realize that for the first time in a long time I feel "normal," more like myself. Until this moment, I was unaware of how very unlike myself I've been feeling. It took the trauma of the freezing cold loft with the broken plumbing for me to come completely unstuck. To start a process of sticking all the pieces back together, correctly assembled. I'm disappointed that I'm not in Vancouver, that my plan hasn't worked out, but I'm also aware that I'm mourning a fantasy.

I want to have the second surgery soon. The part of my intestine that's now on my abdomen, the stoma, will be pulled back into my abdomen, and a pouch will be formed to act as a reservoir. This pouch will then simulate the function of my former colon and my rectum. The remains of my sigmoid colon and my rectum will be removed, and the newly created internal pouch will be attached to my anus. The ultimate goal is for me to end up functioning "normally."

I call the surgeon's office to tell her that I've returned from Vancouver and want the second surgery as soon as possible. I tell Athena's secretary that I'm also still discharging a lot of blood and mucus and experiencing a lot of rectal cramping. Now that there's no waste passing through these areas, they are supposed to heal, but they haven't. I develop deep-breathing techniques to get me through the worst spasms, relaxing my body as much as possible to ride the wave of pain. But it's happening more and more frequently and has become incapacitating at times. Athena's goddess-secretary is very sympathetic but can't get me a surgical date until April. They have a very large number of cancer surgeries scheduled, and of course, these have to take priority.

The endocrinologist's office has a cancellation, so they get me in right away. When I arrive, a medical student leads me into the examining room with his chart and starts asking questions. He's excited about how well I'm fulfilling all the symptoms he's been taught to expect from patients with adrenal failure. He especially likes the blacking out in the Vancouver loft part. Up until this point in the story, he keeps asking, as I describe my symptoms through December, "Did you faint? Did you faint?" And I assure him that that part is coming. When I finish describing all of my symptoms in detail—leaden muscles, joint pain, exhaustion, headaches, and abdominal cramping, he observes, "You know, you sound like you read the textbook." He says this with a smile but clearly is a little bit suspicious.

Irritated, I respond coolly, "No. If I had read the textbook, I would tell you that I have increased thirst and urination. I don't."

He looks taken aback. I smile sweetly. He takes my hand and examines the palm without explanation, simply a "*hmmph*." I want to tell him that, if *he* had read the textbook, he would know that changes in pigmentation generally only occur in primary adrenal failure. As mine was brought on by high-dose steroid treatment, it's considered "secondary" and, as such, is unlikely to produce the dark patches he seems to be looking for. But I bite my tongue. Although it would have been delicious intellectual fun, it likely wouldn't have been a good practical strategy for receiving optimum care.

He calls the specialist in. The doctor wants me to start tapering the steroids again at the beginning of March. Then he'll do some blood tests to see if my adrenal glands are functioning. He doesn't really listen to my concerns about how this might impact me before my next surgery. I've been hoping that there would be some remedy for the extreme exhaustion I'm experiencing. He seems quite unmoved by the fact that my life consists of sleep, pain, and not much else. I read later that, in the letter to my doctor and surgeon, he describes me as "feeling well." I think this happened because I'm so calm and descriptive. He can't seem to reconcile my apparent coherence with the bodily distress I describe.

I read endless articles about biochemistry, developing new theories about my disease process. I apply to a new master's program at York University in Toronto in critical disability studies, and I sign up to speak at conferences in the spring. I spend the rest of my time either writing the early version of this book or sending emails. As I wait for responses about proposals and references from professors and contact from busy friends, my sense of self-worth is based on the number of emails I receive and what their content reveals. My identity becomes indiscernible from my hard drive.

I sink further. Suddenly, I find myself surrounded by dirty laundry. Piles and piles, and I don't know what to do with any of it. So I start to cry, gasping, sobbing, shaking.

Blair walks in. "What's wrong? What's wrong?"

"I don't know. I don't know what to do."

He starts to help me. Patiently picking up each item, asking where we should put it. But I stop him.

"No, no. Don't touch that. I just can't deal with any of this."

So he stops. We go into the other room and watch DVDs and never discuss the incident again. But I can't escape from this overwhelming leaden encasement that is pulling and imprisoning me.

Soon enough, it's time for another hospital pre-surgical education session. This time, it's entirely up to the residents to talk to me and prepare me for the next operation. The first group of three that comes in can't answer any of my questions.

"What is the point of this?" I ask Blair when they leave. "I feel like I know more than they do anyway."

He agrees. "You don't just feel like it, you *do* know more about this than they do. Think about how much they cram into their heads about so many different things. This is all you read about."

Another resident arrives with a checklist. She starts asking me questions. The first ten are about symptoms and how long I've been sick. Then she gets to the mental health section.

"Are you experiencing anxiety?"

"Yes."

"Depression?"

"Yes."

She looks up, with an eyebrow raised, as if wanting more information but not having the appropriate question on her list.

I smile sarcastically. "You can refer back to answers one through ten. Wouldn't you be anxious and depressed?"

"So what do you do?" she asks, barely looking up and completely ignoring my question.

"I'm not doing anything."

"You're on sick leave? Or are you a student?"

"No, I don't have a job. I'm not in school. I'm nothing."

Blair objects to this characterization. "You're a student."

"No. I'm nothing. I tried to go back to my program again in January, but now I've withdrawn twice for being ill; there's no way I'll get back in. I'm not enrolled in anything. I'm not on sick leave for anything. I am nothing."

I'm so tired of sugar-coating everything to make it palatable and digestible. To fit into a tangible category on their charts.

She asks if there's anything currently going on that we haven't covered.

"I have really bad rectal pain, and still lots of bloody mucus that I feel urgency with. Sometimes the spasms are terrible."

"When does it hurt?" she asks.

"All the time," I say.

"Is there anything you do that makes it worse?"

"Moving."

"Okay." She makes a note. "Do you have any other questions?"

"Well, I saw an endocrinologist who wants me to start tapering the steroids now. But if I'm getting surgery in April, I'm just going to have to increase the dose for surgery anyway, right? Because it could be dangerous otherwise, right?"

Much to my surprise, she bursts out, "Yeah! Screw the taper!"

I laugh because it's so unexpected.

She flushes with embarrassment. "That was so unprofessional."

But for me, it's just such a relief that she's willing to be honest and human with me.

She gets up. "I'm going to go talk this through with my senior resident, and I'll come back and let you know what she says."

After Blair and I wait for what feels like an interminable amount of time, I hear her discussing the matter with the senior resident and another student in the hallway. I get impatient and go outside. I pretend not to be listening, as if I just had another question about my surgery occur to me.

Surprised by my sudden appearance and relevant question, they say, "Oh, we were just talking about that!"

Newsflash to doctors and medical students: when you're talking about a patient or, more specifically, about a J-Pouch surgery right outside of an examining room, remember there is potentially an ear on the other side of the door, rapt with attention at your every word.

Then the senior resident starts talking about how I might need to keep my ileostomy for a while. To which I say, "What?" Because the whole point of this surgery is to reverse the ileostomy.

And she says patronizingly, "You know, you have a bag," and pats her abdomen very slowly.

At this point the mini-me in my head surges into combat mode, leaping into kung fu posture and drop-kicking her in the head. As she slams forcefully into the wall, I snap back to the smell of hospital disinfectant to discover that I haven't moved and she is still talking.

I glare at her with full force. "I know what an ileostomy is. The point of this surgery is to reverse it."

"Right, yeah, of course. We just need you to sign this form in case you still need one after. But don't worry, it won't happen. You just have to sign it."

In all, the appointments that day take a total of five hours. By the time we leave, I feel my transformation is complete. I am now J-Pouch. Julie Pouch. Julie Pouch-Devaney. Nobody should ever hear themselves being spoken of in this way. Really amazing doctors have since defended what I overheard in the hallway as necessary "education" for those students, but I still think it's bullshit. I'm either a person or a J-Pouch. There is no middle ground.

By the time we get home, I can barely stumble up the stairs to lie in bed. My head is producing such raging pain that it encases my body in a metal coffin. I can't see or hear. I can barely speak. I'm overwhelmed with nausea. I wonder if I'm having a stroke. I am literally rendered motionless by this overwhelming, suffocating anxiety.

Blair comes into the room. I tell him that I feel like I'm dying.

"Tell my lungs to breathe. Tell them I need air. Tell my stomach to stop heaving. Tell my head to stop to stop to stop. Make it stop."

He quietly places his hands on each piece of my defiant body.

"Stop hurting my Julie. Stop."

Gradually, I start breathing. I learn something new here. Healing is not an enforced act of heroism. There's no health care professional big and strong enough to save me, and no amount of my stoicism and insistence will do it. Healing requires trust and teamwork. It starts with feeling safe, and it can't be done alone.

4. New York in the Spring

I would like to give you the silver branch, the small white
flower, the one word that would protect you from the
grief at the centre of your dream...& become the boat
that would row you back carefully, a flame in two cupped
hands...
> —Margaret Atwood, "Variations on the Word Sleep"

After my complete anxiety-induced body shutdown the day of my hospital
appointments, I realize that I'm going to have to do things differently.
I make a pact with myself: no more computers, no more gym, no more
intellectual exertion, no more organizing anything except for how
many chapters to read in which novel or how long to play mouse with
Willow the kitten. I'm in the bookstore one day when a title jumps out
at me— *When the Body Says No*. It's a book by a Vancouver doctor about
autoimmune diseases. I pick it up and flip it open to the table of contents.
And inexplicably, I start crying. In the bookstore.

I buy the book and read it in one sitting. It confirms everything I've
intuitively known and felt about my illness. The very real physical things
that are happening to my body are related to my life and my emotions. The
book's author, Gabor Maté, clearly has no judgment about this fact. There's

no sense from him that the patients he's writing about are somehow less credible because he sees personality patterns related to their diagnoses. I remember having a moment lying in bed, reading his analysis that patients with colitis tend to be perfectionists, and thinking, *Well, that's not me at all, I've never done anything perfectly once in my whole entire life!*

I burst out laughing. Loudly and raucously, because, if there was ever a definition for perfectionism, I just nailed it with that thought. Lying here, in this bed, laughing to myself, I start to see so clearly how so many things about me that are good qualities, things that are socially praised and supported, are actually deadly when taken to an extreme. So, for example, Dr. Maté talks to one woman with an autoimmune condition who is very successful but always feels like she's not good enough. He points to a building and asks her why she doesn't go and lift it up. She answers that obviously she can't physically pick up a building. And I see his point. So many of the standards I set for myself are just not possible, or even necessarily desirable. And yet I beat myself up harshly when I don't reach them. Although this way of being, when enacted in moderation, can support me achieving lovely and exciting things, in its extreme, it makes me sick.

So I'm immediately won to the idea that I need a psychotherapist who uses this method. I find one who practises near my parents' house. Her name is Grace and she runs chronic illness therapy groups. When I meet her for the first time, I feel this profound sense of relief. When she asks me about my life and what's been happening, I choke up pretty quickly.

"It's okay to cry here, Julie," she says.

She asks me about my future plans.

"Well, I *was* planning to do grad work," I answer bitterly.

And she says, "You will get through this; you will be able to do these things." Then she smiles. She's such a serious person that I believe her. There's no false bubbliness or condescension about her. Just a quiet, calm assuredness.

We talk about the fact that just because physical symptoms can be caused by emotions, it doesn't mean that these symptoms are any less valid, or dangerous. I tell her that I now believe this psychotherapy process is essential to my recovery. I'm committing, and I don't take any kind of commitment lightly.

Date: Sat, 6 Mar 2004 21:46:37 -0800 (PST)
From: Julie Devaney
Subject: a final digest of the bulk barn variety

poof!
that was me. I vapourized. disapparated.

I'm turning off my computer and not turning it back on for the next couple of months. "Impossible!" I hear you all cry. And you're probably right. But it is a noble endeavour. One which suggests that I might actually get better this time.

So the final updates are as follows...in order of "news"

1. My next surgery is scheduled for sometime in April. I don't actually know when it will be. I'm the first in line for non-cancer surgery. Officially, I'm considered "elective." I can't understand why all of you aren't electing for this surgery. Surely there must be something fab about it otherwise I wouldn't be "electing" to do it.

I had a five hour pre-op appt. at the hospital last Monday. There I met pharmacy students who knew less about my meds than me and med students who were sent instead of doctors and who didn't know which surgery I was having but really wanted to draw a picture. I'm not kidding. I gently tried to correct them to clarify matters but they were having none of it. I had a nurse who said "that's impossible" twice when I told her about something that *happened* after my last surgery. Then the students came back after having a loud conversation in the hallway that I presume they thought I wasn't listening to and spoke very very slowly to clear up "my" confusion. Patronizing little shits. 5 hours. Finally they sent a doctor after 4 hours and 45 minutes who agreed with everything I had been saying all along, *corrected* my chart notes then wrote it down separately for me so that I could repeat "her" opinion to my endocrinologist and to the anaesthesiologist before my surgery. She complained about cutbacks and then said, "You shouldn't have to advocate for yourself like this, but you seem to be good at it."

I left the hospital with a migraine that lasted for three days. The students and nurse should be eternally grateful to Blair because if he hadn't taken the day off of work to come with me we would all be in hospital. Them in the trauma unit, me in the psych ward.

2. I need to relax...hospitals are bad for my health and I apparently could be in for ten days this time. I need to prepare. So, I've decided that I'm giving up suffering for Lent. This works well because the surgery will likely be around Easter...Indulgence, indulgence, then more indulgence. No computers and nothing that smells remotely like work.

3. I'm not in Vancouver. Sorry for anyone that's so out of the loop that they still think that I am. I was there for about 36 hours and I don't want to talk about it.

I'm still answering the phone.

For those in distant lands snail mail is your only option.

So poof! This is really it. The Cyber-Julie is gone.

•

I now organize my weeks entirely around my Wednesday therapy group. I read every book on Grace's recommended chronic illness reading list. A few of them are actually about being sick, but most of them are about developing new emotional skills. The thing I find most compelling in this process is the idea that I can just be curious about myself. I learn to give myself a break and see how I'm feeling without worrying so much about why or if I think I *should* be feeling that way. I discover connections between my physical pain and specific emotions like fear and insecurity. Every week, I haul out pieces from the deep recesses of my psyche and the surface interactions of day-to-day life. I tell my stories, express my feelings to the group, and with Grace's guidance, we talk it through. I start the process of moving up and through to the other side.

And in the safety of Grace's group, I have my first ever temper tantrum. I can't even remember what it started off being about, something seemingly minor. But it soon turned into me yelling and stomping my feet.

"It's not fair! I'm doing everything I'm supposed to do! I just want to get better! It's all just *so* unfair."

As Grace encourages me, I destroy her tissue box that sits in the centre of our group's circle. I kick over the stand it was on. When I sit back down, I say, "That was my first tantrum."

"I know," says Grace. She's smiling, but her eyes are serious.

When I get home, I ask my mother, "When I was a little kid, did I have temper tantrums?"

"No." She answers immediately, without even having to think about it.

"Not ever?" I press. "Not even when I was, like, two?"

"No," she says. "You were such a good baby. You were never any trouble."

It's so unbelievable to me. When I made the claim in Grace's group, I thought I might just have been misremembering my childhood. But here my mum confirms it.

As I continue to work in group, I discuss my self-image issues. The emotional pain of feeling like my body in this state is disgusting, repulsive. Gradually, my harsh self-judgments lift. I would never think these things about other people. I learn to apply some of the generosity I offer others to myself. And then one day, I find myself in the bathroom, looking in the mirror, and actually admiring my stoma. Hanging through clear plastic, unashamedly making its power and purpose known to the world. I notice how as I inhale, the stoma expands with my breath, and as I exhale, it becomes small again. I watch this process with a new fascination, amazed that I can actually see my intestine work. The tissue that forms the stoma is the identical tissue that forms our tongues. My intestines are defiantly sticking their tongue out at the world. Rudely sputtering their waste, their life force, *in your general direction.* I realize that it's not directing its defiance *toward* me, as I'd once thought. It's expressing my irreverent rebellion to the world.

My energy level improves massively. I go to visit Joanne in New York. I leave on a Thursday and come back on Tuesday, just to make sure I don't miss my group with Grace. The world is colourful and bright. It's such a contrast—everything looks different with energy. The bleak, grey cloud is lifting. We walk around, we hang out with Joanne's friends, we eat lots of good food. I return to Toronto to prepare for surgery number two.

Every week in Grace's group, we begin with five minutes of meditation. But every time I close my eyes, I panic. I ultimately keep my eyes lowered and focused on a spot on the carpet. Whatever visual stimuli I'm getting from having my eyes open, gazing upon the feet and carpet fibres in front of me, is pure peace and calm compared to the chaos inside of me. My April surgery is quickly approaching.

When it arrives, we head to the hospital just like last time. I go to my room, where a nurse starts my IV. They take me to the operating theatre while my mum and Blair sit in my room. I'm scared this time, and really *feeling* it in a way I've never allowed myself to before. But it's a brand-new experience of fear. Instead of resisting it, I feel really calm — the terror swells up like an ocean's tide, meeting me and recessing, meeting me and recessing. I learn that I can be okay while feeling terrified. The anaesthetic kicks in and I fall asleep.

5. Dawn Escape

And now, I'm in the recovery room.

Lying on my stretcher, I discover the April of T.S. Eliot's "The Waste Land." "...the cruellest month, breeding / Lilacs out of the dead land, mixing / Memory and desire..."

I can't feel my body but feel very present in my mind, so I ask the nurse, "Is it still there? Can you look?"

I am terrified that the surgery didn't work out, but I'm incapable of checking myself in my highly drugged state.

She lifts my gown. "Yes, it is."

I don't believe her, so I ask another nurse. I need a second opinion. "Can you please look?"

So she looks and agrees.

But I'm still not sure if I believe them. I ask what happened, why the surgery didn't go as planned, where the doctor is, and why no one is explaining what happened to me. They don't know.

Then I'm alone again. So I start crying, loudly and unashamedly. Gasping and shaking, I'm fading in and out of consciousness, but I sense that a lot of time is passing. Patients move on either side of me but I'm still lying here. Every time I wake up I'm still crying, and I don't know if I've stopped crying even in my sleep. This moment is immortalized in my chart notes with the words "Patient weepy." They encourage me to push the button on my pain pump. It's making me feel really woozy and it's also not changing the fact that no one has explained to me why there is still a bag on my abdomen following five hours of surgery that was supposed to get rid of it.

One of the nurses asks another nurse over my head, "What's the matter with *her*?"

"Oh, she's just embarrassed because she still has a bag."

"No, I'm not!" I explode.

The ghost of Julie has a megaphone in hand. When on the outside I am calmly and dispassionately addressing medical professionals, the ghost inside screams and curses, the bell of her megaphone full on in their faces. Now, on the stretcher in the recovery room I am possessed by my own ghost.

In this moment I accept myself and everything about me without question. It really is the rest of the world that is irreconcilably flawed.

"That's not it at all! I've been in and out of hospitals for two years. I'm twenty-four! This is supposed to be over, and all I know is that it isn't but no one has come to tell me why, or what happens next, or anything!"

The nurse looks contrite. "Yes, okay, we'll find someone to talk to you."

I'm still fading in and out and sobbing. The nurses intermittently come back and apologize that they don't know what's going on and they've put in lots of calls to the doctors but no one is responding.

Finally a young man appears at my side and introduces himself as doctor something.

I am immediately suspicious.

"Are you a resident?" I ask.

"Yes."

"Were you even in on my operation?"

"Well, no."

I remember my pre-operation appointment with the guessing med students and the residents suggesting based on textbooks what the details of my surgery might be, and I realize that I might actually kill him if that's what he intends to do.

So for his own safety, I say, "I really don't want to talk to you then. I'm looking for a real doctor that actually knows what happened."

He is very nice and probably relieved because he can accurately report that he tried to talk to me but "the patient refused."

So he says, "I understand."

And off he goes.

At some point, the nurses change shifts and I can tell that time is passing again. I recognize Doris, the nurse from my first operation. As she walks past me, I call out to her.

"Doris?"

She turns around in surprise.

"Yes?"

"Do you remember me? I was here in October."

And she looks at another nurse and laughs, "Do I remember her?" As if it's absurd that she possibly could.

"Your cat's called Harry Houdini and mine's Willow Rosenberg, remember?"

"Oh yeah, yeah, I remember!"

The world is still very foggy, but I want to tell her that she's in chapter 9. "I'm writing a book. You're in my book."

Excited, she wants to know if it's available and when she can buy it. I indicate to my still-immobile body that the story is ongoing. Another nurse tells me that my respiration is a "two." I don't know what this means, but apparently the value of my breathing is inadequate. I suggest that maybe if I had some information about the state of my body, I could start breathing normally.

She asks me to rate my pain between one and ten. I close my eyes and breathe deeply, carefully considering the intensity of my pain.

"Eight point five."

Impatiently, she repeats the same rote I've heard a thousand times before.

"A ten is the *worst* pain you've ever had. How much *pain* are you in?"

I close my eyes again, calling down to my abdomen, asking for an answer.

"Eight point five."

"There's no way your pain could be that high!"

I roll my eyes, thinking, *Yes I just faked bowel surgery.*

"Well, we can't move you out of the recovery room until you rate your pain lower."

"How low does it need to be?"

"I don't know. Three or four maybe."

"Okay, it's three or four. Can I go to my room now?"

Finally, recognizing the absurdity of the situation, she softens, agreeing that I must be in a lot of pain and encouraging me to push the button on the morphine pump.

She returns a little while later.

"How are you feeling?"

As my ghost finally leaves my body, she whispers, *Like I was pinned down, knocked out, sliced up, and stapled back together. Like I was lied to. Beaten and bruised into submission.*

But the spirit leaves me before my mouth opens to respond, so I just say, "Fine."

When we approach the doorway to my room, the thread of composure snaps. Again, I burst into tears.

"What? What is it?" asks the now sympathetic nurse.

"I don't want to tell them." I say. "They don't know that I need another operation; I don't want to tell them."

"They probably know," she tells me.

And she's right. As I'm wheeled back into Room 1402, Bed 2, Blair and my mum are standing with comforting smiles. Athena, the surgeon, phoned the waiting room just before going into her next surgery, so my mum had known everything, all along. But no one had allowed her to come into the recovery room to see me. My five hours of hell could have been avoided. But the part that still breaks my heart is that because my surgery took way too long and I was so ridiculously long in recovery, Mum and Blair had to wait more than ten hours to see me.

Usually, when I remember scenes throughout my life where I was truly panicking, they replay in Technicolor, as if everything in the world becomes important: every shade, every detail, every fragment highlighted. But when I remember lying on that stretcher in the recovery room, I can't see anything. I am suffocating as the world bleeds away. The giant dusty stage curtains from the school gymnasium are weighing down on my face, in all their eighties-velour glory. Drowning between the creases of medical words. Words that describe everything, yet mean nothing. The terms that swim like tepid soup through my mouth and nose, banal as they pass one by one, but incapacitating as they accumulate into a monsoon after two long, unbearable years.

. . . ulcerative colitis. Severe. Pancolonic. Mild. Distal. Crohn's. Severe. Refractory. Steroid-dependent ulcerative colitis. Masked. Subtotal colectomy. End-ileostomy. Temporary.

Disintegrating rectum. Loop ileostomy. Functional. Blood. Test test test. Chemotherapeutic agent. Toxic therapy. Blood blood blood blood. Bleeding rectum. Disintegrating.

I have a meditation CD with me for this hospitalization. I listen to it before I go to sleep. Through the night, I wake up and realize that I have my period. I buzz the nurse and ask her if she can pass me the pads I've packed in my bag. She's got headphones on, dangling around her neck. I can hear the base and percussion resonating from the music that's still pumping through them as she talks to me. I'd guess her age at mid-twenties. She looks around under the sheet, to see how much I'm bleeding, and she tells me that I can't use my own, that the hospital has special ones because of the catheters in my urethra and anus. She waves her hand dismissively and says she'll come back, but she doesn't. So I lie there soaking in my menstrual blood, waiting.

The worst part is that the whole time, there's an incredibly kind and caring nurse taking care of my roommate. She offers to rub her back. She recommends positions for her to lie in. She checks on her frequently, speaking to her in a soft, soothing voice. At one point when she's about to leave, I call out to her and ask if she can help with the situation with my period.

"You'll have to page your nurse," she says in a really annoyed tone.

Looking back, I can only guess that it's the other nurse she's angry with for not doing her job. But, at the time, it feels like a slap in the face.

When I drift back to sleep I have a terrifying nightmare. I'm a little kid, and I'm being chased by a man through a house on a mountain. The dream is so real. As I run away from him, there's a really horrible taste in my mouth, and I know he's done something to me but I don't know what. When I wake up, I'm shaking and crying, and the taste is still in my mouth. It's the most real-feeling nightmare I've ever had, and the bitter, sour aftertaste is seeping through my body. The smells and physical sensations of the dream are still present in the room. I'm disoriented and shaking. I buzz the nurses' station.

A nurse arrives and I ask her to sit with me, to hold my hand. "I just had a really terrible dream and I don't want to be alone."

It's a different nurse this time, probably in her fifties. She looks down at me with a patronizing smile and says, "It's just a dream; you'll be fine." And leaves.

I stay awake for the rest of the night, stiff, frozen in terror.

The doctor, the fellow with the round, round, brown watery eyes, appears by my bed the next morning. Scared. Hollow. Alone. No team of students with clipboards. *She's not an exhibit any more, folks. This, this is serious.*

"You were disintegrating."

His eyes search mine, as if for a sign. *What does the soul of a Disintegrating Woman look like?*

I was invisible on the gurney. Then when I yelled out in the recovery room, I was a basket case. He searches my eyes, the eyes of the Disintegrating Woman.

The doctor with the brown eyes has seen pieces of me that I have not — that hopefully I never will. Yet, I was unconscious while he voyeuristically observed the cutting, the reconstruction. When I am simply a mass of cells, a Body, there is no need for clarity on the notion that The Disease is the threat, the enemy to be eradicated. Dealing with The Person is a much more complex challenge.

I look back coldly, directly, and push out words like light bulb shards into his warm, brown eyes.

He begs. "It was just so, so diseased."

"I know."

"It was almost disintegrating."

"I know."

We both wish he could be The Hero. He wants to save me. I want to be saved. But we are both drowning, clutching, gasping. He in impotence, me in fear. And so he goes away. "Nothing to learn here, kids."

A few hours later, Athena comes in looking sympathetic.

"I heard you're mad at me."

"What? No!"

I can't imagine how the events of the last day and a half have been spun to lead her to that conclusion. First, I was mad at the nurses for their demeaning projections about my bag. Then I was generally angry that no one was telling me what was going on or being even remotely nurturing and sympathetic. Finally, I was furious when I found out that although Athena had phoned my mum in the surgical waiting room, so my mum knew exactly what happened the whole time, they wouldn't let Mum in to see me.

"Once we got in there, we just couldn't attach the pouch. The tissue was too damaged."

"I'm not really that surprised," I tell her. "I was in so much rectal pain for the past few months. I was just scared you found a tumour or something."

"No, no, nothing like that. The next procedure will only take forty-five minutes. We've already built the internal J-Pouch with your small intestine, it just needs a chance to heal. Then we can do the closure surgery where we remove your stoma and attach your bowel to the J-Pouch in June." I don't know why I should care how long the next procedure will take. It seems kind of immaterial. But then I try to move and I learn what the after-effects of five hours of laparoscopic bowel cutting and manipulation feel like.

I go home and a week passes. And then a night where nothing passes. Blair and I stay up all night watching the bag to see if it will start to fill up. I'm in tons of pain. I phone the ward, the nurse tells me to come into emergency and that Kathy and Nicole, the specialist therapy nurses, will come down and meet me when their shift starts at 6:30 a.m. Being driven down Yonge Street in the pre-dawn dark, I am exhausted from not sleeping, nauseated from painkillers. My senses are thread-bare.

We arrive and are immediately seen by an emergency department resident. He doesn't want to inspect the site in case it leaks on him. Seriously.

He's all like, "Just keep the bag on." He screws his face up.

I laugh at him. "It's okay, I'm not planning to take it off until the enterostomal therapy nurses get here. They're going to fix my stoma. Kathy and Nicole know I'm coming; they're supposed to meet me down here."

He smirks and snickers, like we're sharing a joke, but the reality is I'm laughing because I think he's pathetic. I'm not remotely embarrassed; I feel very confident in this moment that he's the one with the problem. He's training to be a doctor and he's worried about seeing poo and intestines. In the meantime, somewhere, in the gallows of the hospital, a team of surgical residents is using their supersonic senses to detect that I am here. The emerg resident is just leaving when I hear their thundering steps in rhythm and see their white coats billowing toward my booth in the ER.

The senior resident is wearing loud, clicking high heels and a brisk, clipped smile. It's not her fault that she has the same name as a woman in Vancouver who I hate, but the shoes are definitely her fault. She immediately starts hammering me with question after question in a booming gym-teacher voice, flanked by messy-haired, just-woke-up med students on either side. Without actually listening to the answers, she orders a battery of tests and admits me to stay until the next day.

When the nurse comes back, I tell her, "I don't need these tests, I just need to see Kathy and Nicole."

Clearly sharing my opinion, she looks gleeful when she responds, "Well, you can refuse."

Kathy and Nicole arrive and gently and sweetly fix what they describe as a "mechanical problem" with my stoma. As they work, technologists arrive with orders to take me to various places for various tests. I apologize to each one, explaining that I don't think the tests are necessary, so I'm not going. I tell Kathy and Nicole my frustrations.

"I've been telling health care professionals over and over since *November* how much pain I was in! And then, in *April*, when they cut me open, they're all shocked to find my flesh disintegrating. But I knew."

Kathy says, "Of course you knew. It was inside of you."

The ER nurses page the residents again, so I can talk to them and ask them to discharge me, but they don't come this time. Hospital pages are apparently less compelling than supersonic senses. A nurse brings me a form to sign that I am leaving against the doctors' orders. I feel powerful, and considering what has transpired, this feeling is somewhat remarkable. The sheer force of my illness made everything solid in my life melt into air. Now, everything that had disintegrated suddenly becomes solid.

Dawn happened while we were in the dank and faceless ER. The space that exists beyond geographical borders, the land of latex and disinfectant. It happened sometime between my first "refusal of treatment" and the moment I discharged myself from the ER "against medical advice." In that place furiously buried between my brows, between fear and defiance, in my simple act of resistance. But I don't know that morning has broken until we are in the car, driving home. And then I finally fall asleep.

In the coming weeks, the stoma continues to work normally.

At the end of May, Blair and I take a road trip to Winnipeg. It's essentially our honeymoon because we haven't taken a trip together since we got married. The night before my birthday, we stay in this awesome place on the north shore of Lake Superior. Our room is on a little piece of land that juts out into the lake, so we're surrounded by water. I'm remembering the events of the past six weeks as we sit on the edge of the lake on my twenty-fifth birthday, and I write them down in my notebook. As the waves come crashing in, I just feel this intense sense of calm, of peace, of having made it to the other side. Blair and I have a perfect little holiday.

When we get to Winnipeg, I present at an academic conference on disability studies. My essay is about the treatment I got from Mitzi, Snot-Face, and the graduate advisor in Vancouver. A woman in the audience is editing an anthology about women and chronic illness. She approaches me afterwards, and ultimately my story of academic mistreatment becomes a chapter in her academic book. It's so indescribably amazing to not only be heard, but also to be acknowledged and praised for sharing this narrative and producing an analysis. One of my friends from undergrad is living in Winnipeg now, so we stay with her and her partner and son. We stay up late, just chatting and hanging out.

Blair and I love long drives, and we have a really fun time going home, meeting moose and otters along the way. When we get back to Toronto, my sister and mum, both of whom worried about the wisdom of me going on a road trip at this stage in my recovery, are thrilled and relieved to see the new colour in my cheeks and the sparkle in my eyes.

6. Closure

Less than a month later, I have my final surgery. It's June 30, 2004. My terror is overwhelming this time. I do *not* want to be hospitalized again. But it's a trade-off because, even more than that, I want all of this to be over, and this surgery promises to be the end.

The porters are pushing my stretcher into the elevator. We're heading down for operation number three. This one is called "closure." I've already written hundreds of pages at this point, spooling out the trauma into neat lines of typed words. And I panic. There's nowhere to type. There's no sea of beautiful words swimming around me, waiting to be splashed on the page, inviting me to dive in. There's just me, a sheet, and a gown. And people pushing me. Pushing me with my consent. Pushing me in my horror and vulnerability to surgery number three. So I begin furiously typing in my head. Moving in and out of the scene, between narrator and subject. I picture the boy on the package of baking soda, holding the package with the boy on the package, holding the package with the picture of the boy.... I'm eight years old sitting in the laundry room, staring at the box. I'm in the elevator.

And I'm spinning. In and out and in. Writer and subject. On the page, in the scene, in my head, in my body. My head wants to see what happens next, what interesting moment I can record, which new character will appear to be mocked. And my body just wants it to stop. Here. In the elevator, on the sheet, in the gown. Stop. My eyes see the scratches on the ceiling. The things you never see standing in an elevator. And I think of the clever things I can say about the legions of patients flat on our backs lying here. Trying to claw our way out. But it's not funny. I'm panicking because nothing funny is happening. There's no keyboard, nowhere to type, and nothing funny is happening at all. I don't know what happens next.

When I wake up, I'm in the recovery room and I'm gagging. A nurse is attaching a bag of morphine to my IV pole.

"I can't have that without the other medication first," I tell her.

"What?"

She looks confused. I explain that, if she looks at my chart, she'll see that I need another medication to allay the symptoms I get from taking that much morphine by itself.

The nurse leaves, finds out there's another med ordered, and comes back with it.

"And I need a pump for the morphine," I explain, "because I can't take that much at once or I'll vomit; I need really small doses."

She's getting angry at this point, "Well, that's all that's ordered. No one ordered you a pump!"

"Well, can you please get me some Gravol then? I know that that much morphine is going to make me sick, and I'm already really nauseated."

"All I have is this morphine. Do you want it or not?" She's standing over me with one hand on her hip.

"Um, well, okay then. But could you please find out about getting me a pump?"

She administers the morphine and storms off.

Whenever I'm in a dire situation, there's a checklist in my head of "appropriate" versus "authentic" reactions. When I choose authenticity, I get branded as hysterical. But when I choose what I decide is "appropriate," it calls the depth of my agony into question. Still, these fake calm and measured responses allow me to manage the situation and advocate for myself. It's always a toss-up determining which path people will respond to best. I doze off, and when I wake up, I'm gagging again. I call out to another nurse, "Can you please find me some Gravol?"

She goes to talk to the first nurse I've been dealing with. They're only a couple of feet away from me and I can see them. The first nurse writes something down, points to me, and then hands it to the other nurse.

Then she walks over and says to me, "How much of this are you taking at home?"

I'm confused. "Gravol?"

"No!" she says. "Morphine."

"None!" I can't believe she's accusing me of being a drug addict. Especially considering I'm asking for less medication, not more. How does that even make sense? I tell her, "This is my third surgery in nine months. There's a protocol I've figured out with the pain specialist and my surgeon and my endocrinologist about what meds I take when. And for some reason the orders in the chart are wrong."

I don't want a repeat of my previous five-hour stint in the recovery room, so I smile calmly and sweetly at the end of this and say, "It's fine, I feel fine, just take me to the floor and I'll get it sorted out up there."

When we get upstairs and I repeat my request, the floor nurse says, "It's just closure surgery. We don't usually give pumps for that."

He's a male nurse, probably in his mid-forties. By now, the first dose of morphine has worn off and I'm getting really grumpy, "*Just closure surgery*? How many times have *you* had closure surgery?"

He looks defensive. "We have closure surgeries on the ward all the time."

"No, not your patients, *you*. How many times have *you* recovered from a closure operation on your own body?"

"I don't have the kind of problems you do!" He storms out and I never see him again. Another nurse comes back and tells me she's going to page the residents.

A surgical resident called Bruno marches in and asks to see my surgical site. He's got two residents with him, one on each side. I tentatively lift my gown, not really clear what this has to do with sorting out my meds. He sticks his finger right onto the surgical site and pokes hard. I scream.

"It's just surgical pain," he declares, and then leaves with his little friends trailing out behind him.

I look up at my mum and Blair.

"Mum," I say. "I need you to leave."

She's shocked. "Why?"

"Because I really need to swear and it's going to upset you."

My mother can't stand foul language, specifically the f-word, used in front of her. So I respect this and keep my language fairly clean around her. But, today, after she's witnessed the outrageous behaviour of Bruno, the resident, she looks at me and says emphatically, "Go ahead."

We're temporarily in a private room until my actual assigned space becomes available. So I yell, "That fucking little arrogant piece of shit! He just stuck his fucking finger into my surgical site to make some kind of point! The power-tripping asshole! He poked my fucking surgical site!"

Blair goes marching down to Athena's office. He tells them what's going on, and before he even gets back, a nurse has pushed a morphine pump into my room.

When the nurses change shifts, I get the most amazing team. For the rest of my stay, I have lovely, nurturing people taking care of me. I tell them what happened with Bruno and they're furious. Apparently he's been awful to them the whole time he's been training there.

One nurse even offers to wheel me down to the ombuds office to make a complaint.

On my last day, my favourite nurse comes to remove the draining tube from my surgical site. She rushes in and says, "Let's do this quickly before someone comes to take your pump back!"

She's so caring and amazing. She says, "Okay, push the button now and then we'll wait a few minutes. Let me know when you feel it."

I wait for the sensation of the morphine.

"It's working," I tell her.

"Okay, breathe deeply," she says.

I begin inhaling and exhaling into my belly. She gently slides the draining pump out of my surgical site, firmly applies gauze, and tapes it shut. I don't feel a thing.

The porter who I've been chatting with every time he changes my garbage bag arrives with orders to move me to another room. My nurse is still there, and they discuss how ridiculous and disruptive that is considering I'm leaving in a few hours. They team up and refuse to move me. When Blair and my mum come to pick me up, we all agree that this hospital stay has ended very well.

Later, I tell Athena's goddess-secretary, "Bruno is an asshole."

When I go to my follow-up appointment, she tells me, "I told Athena what you said about Bruno." She stage-whispers. "That's he's an *asshole*. And we both agree, if Julie says that about him, he must have done something really awful."

I don't quite get her meaning at first. Anyone who's spent any amount of time with me knows that I have no qualms about calling people such names as I feel are appropriate. But I guess I've always been so polite, accommodating, and easygoing with Athena and her secretary that they take it seriously when I take a stand. Athena encourages me to put my complaint in writing for her and other surgeons, but somehow I just never find it in myself to do it. I still occasionally look him up on the Internet to see where he's working and if other people have complained about him. But, mostly, I just fantasize about unexpectedly meeting him in a dark alley on a dark night. It wouldn't end well for him.

7. Alight

So it turns out that July is, in fact, the cruellest month, and August is just that tiny bit crueller. I spend most of the summer of 2004 in bed. After my closure surgery in June, the recovery is brutal. I end up back in hospital with a bowel blockage where scar tissue has actually adhered my bowel closed. When I get to the emergency room, I tell them, "I have a bowel blockage right here."

Actually, it's more like I gasp this information at them as I practically collapse into a chair. I point at the spot on my abdomen where my stoma was closed. They get me a stretcher to lie down on until there's a booth available.

The emergency room doctor immediately orders the morphine. The type that works best for me is called Dilaudid. As the nurse injects the dose into my IV, I feel an unbelievable sense of relief wash over my body. When she leaves, I start singing to Blair, "Dilaudid, Dilaudid, put your hands all over my body." To the tune of Madonna's "Erotic." We giggle. It's funny because I can honestly say I don't do these things specifically to entertain Blair. That song just pours out of me before I've even considered it. Sometimes I feel like I think things *after* they come out of my mouth.

The surgical resident comes and orders tests. I get carted into the endo-scopy unit and meet the loveliest young female technologist I've ever had.

"Ohhh, you've got a blockage?" she asks sympathetically. "Are you going to be able to get on the table?"

She gently helps me get up, and I ask what she needs to do. She explains that she's going to put a small tube into my anus to inject dye and then put contrast dye into my veins. Then she's going take an image. Unbelievably, none of this is remotely painful or scary. She chats about pleasant things to distract me while she's doing the inserting of tubes and injecting of dyes.

An hour later, the surgical resident comes back and points at the exact same spot on my abdomen I'd pointed at an hour earlier and pronounces, "You have a bowel blockage right there…"

He shows me the images from the elaborate dye process—the ultimate lie-detector test. They admit me and it takes another five days before the blockage fully resolves itself, thankfully without any more surgery.

They discharge me with more pain meds, but every time I try to taper them, I start having withdrawal side effects. I'm constantly nauseated, and now I'm having really bad leg and abdominal cramping every time I lower the dose. So I have an idea. What readily available substance provides pain relief and improves appetite?

I phone my friend Scotty from high school and ask if he can bring some pot over. His source is a really long walk from my parents' house and he smokes the whole way over. So even though his tolerance would normally be a lot higher than mine, we're on a pretty level playing field by the time he arrives. No one's home. This is by coincidence rather than by design—I haven't hidden my plan from Blair or my family. But for some reason, Scotty and I feel the need to sit on the deck behind the giant pine tree in my parents' backyard as if we're still teenagers.

We're walking back into the house, laughing really hard about silly things, when I feel myself hitting the floor. I'm on my hands and knees, and my face is going up and down into the tile. It's really dark, and Scotty has his hand on my shoulder.

"Julie, Julie. Are you all right?"

I feel like I'm being pulled out of a really lovely, peaceful place and I'm resistant at first. Then I'm getting up and saying to Scotty, "What happened?"

He yells, "You were breakdancing, man!"

It's hard to describe how hilarious we find this.

"Breakdancing? That's awesome!"

We really are having an amazing time and giggle endlessly about my newfound capacities as we re-enact the scene.

"So then you went down like this, and I was like this..."

"Like this?"

Our mock breakdancing scene is even funnier than the original.

I figure out later that the combination of the meds still in my system and my undernourishment probably caused a seizure, but obviously at the time, we were too high to realize that this is a problem. I've never actually asked a medical professional why such a thing would happen, but seeing as it never happened again, I don't think much about it.

Three weeks after the blockage, I'm mostly off of the meds, and I start a new master's program in Toronto.

I love my program, but it really is too soon to be back in school. I push and push myself and—unsurprisingly—become very ill. Now we're back to that part in the story where I go to school one day, teach undergraduates the next day, and then go back to bed.

Blair and I moved into our own apartment as soon as I got my student loan, and I start looking for a GP in our new neighbourhood. I find a young woman at a clinic a short walk away from us who is accepting patients. The first time I see her, I take Blair with me as backup. She looks straight at me and says something to the effect of, "You know you have the right to be alone in your health care appointments."

I love that she says this. I explain, "He's with me because I've had really traumatic incidents with doctors I've never met before and I want him with me."

She looks completely unfazed about this.

"Oh," she says. "Well, that's okay then."

We immediately get along. She keeps track of all my specialists and everything I tell her about my history. She advocates for me, getting referrals when I need them. And when I ask a question that she doesn't know the answer to, she says, "Huh, I have no idea. Let me look into it and get back to you."

It's such an incredible relief. No words could have made me feel safer. I'm profoundly comforted by her ability to be human and honest—and assured by the fact that she's always reading and checking and rechecking before she suggests anything complicated.

I also find a naturopath in our new neighbourhood. She's actually someone I've known through friends for ages, but I didn't realize she'd become a naturopath. She's calm and smart and great and clearly doesn't blame me for being ill. Her name is Alina. Instead of loading me with piles of weird diet sheets, she suggests that I try different things slowly and gives me lots of intriguing and yummy recipes. I've hardly been able to digest anything since the "closure" surgery, so her suggestions are all great. In the meantime, I'm still dependent on the steroids for my adrenal function. Athena finds me a new endocrinologist who's going to help me with my adrenal problem. She tends to personality-match me with her colleagues and promises me about this doctor that I'll really like her. "You two will get along for sure."

The endocrinologist's resident is intrigued when I come in with a protocol for re-activating my adrenal glands from Alina, my naturopath. With the endocrinologist's approval, the resident prescribes the necessary dosages and orders the necessary tests. Over the course of that year, in a great feat of cooperation between open-minded health care professionals and my very wise new naturopath, my adrenal tests in the hospital lab go from a result of "not functioning" to "fully functioning," without any steroids at all.

But my bowel continues to cause me constant pain and distress. In April 2005, at the end of the school year, Blair and I take a trip to Cuba. It's a disaster. I'm so sick and thin and feeling so weak all the time. I have a migraine the first couple of days we're there, so we stay inside watching HBO movies while I vomit and weep. I finally start to feel well enough to take the short walk to the beach and enjoy the water. As I'm lying there, I realize, in a different way than I ever have before, that I just need to take care of myself. It doesn't matter if I finish my courses at school, it doesn't matter if I have to put off plans for another year. For right now, all my focus just needs to be about me — gradually nurturing myself back to health.

In a really basic way, I decide that it's up to me to heal. It's not the same thing as saying it's *my fault* when I'm sick. I think there are plenty of reasons to feel unwell when coping with the dysfunction of the world. There are lots of scientific reasons why some of us are more biologically predisposed to sensitivity too. But, to me, all of these things add up to the same conclusion. This is the body I have, this is the environment I live in, so what can I do for myself to make it easier to be here?

8. Am I Zero Yet?

We get back from Cuba, and soon enough it's summertime. I'm thin for the first time in my life. Like visible hip bones and jutting-out ribs kind of thin. And I love it. Every time someone compliments me on my new rakishness, I attempt to shame them with comments like, "Yeah, I heard Kate-Moss-heroin-chic was hot this year. And you know me, anything for fashion." The fact that I achieved this body through three bowel surgeries and a resulting year of starvation appalls me. The fact that I like it horrifies me even more. When I walk into the grocery store, young men stumble over each other to help me. Fashionistas in clothing shops where they used to ignore me want to dress me. Thirteen-year-old boys do skateboarding tricks on the sidewalk and look to see if I saw them. I laugh that I literally am twice their age. And this tips me off, jars me out of my starved reverie. I stare at that image looking back at me in the mirror of the H&M dressing room. I have regressed back through puberty.

To my GP's horror, I'm so anemic that I need a blood transfusion. She's been giving me regular iron injections, so there's no good explanation for this. She finds me a hematologist at the local hospital.

No one has yet been able to explain the severity of my anemia, and I can't help wondering if it's related to my extreme weight loss. I was never this anemic with the colitis, even when I was constantly losing lots of blood.

When I explain to the hematologist how much weight I've lost, he looks disbelieving. He says, "You must've been really big."

I'm shocked and insulted, but I just sort of smile back uncomfortably. I don't remember being *really big*, as he puts it. Sure, I had as many body-hating feelings as the next woman. But I just don't objectively think that at any point in my life, no matter how much I weighed, if anyone said, "Hey, which one's Julie?" someone would've responded, "You know, the really big one." Kind of chubby, maybe, round and cute, possibly, but not *really big*. At times like this, I want to bring back my favourite sarcastic phrase of 1992. *Way to be, doctor, way to be.* It's like his brain divides women into two categories: thin ones who are attractive and appropriate and *fit in*, and fat ones who are marginal, extreme, and unruly. So he seems unable to grasp the idea that there could be anything problematic for my health in the thinness of this socially acceptable body before him. More nurses than I could possibly ever imagine express jealousy when weighing me. And this type of envious commentary continues from all manner of other women, including comments about how, while, of course, they would never want to go through what I went through, just a little bit of bowel disease wouldn't be so bad. "Hahahaha, just kidding," they quickly add. Appalling as their sentiments are, I can hardly blame them, since I secretly smirk with glee at every sighting of a new rib bone peeking out of my back.

I can't say with certainty that the thinness created the anemic break-down, but with even less treatment five years later, and a body weight sitting comfortably midway between its previous extremes, my iron levels are stable and easily managed. When I picture my body at that time, it's almost as if I was hibernating within myself. Shrinking from the outside world to preserve my energy and to hide. Like a computer or printer in energy-conserve mode: blank screen, orange light flashing. People have heart problems when they gain too much weight because their blood pressure increases as their heart has to keep up with all the extra blood circulating to further reaches of flesh. Maybe as I shrank, my heart just kept getting slower, pressure sinking, and my blood just couldn't be bothered to keep its oxygen and iron levels up. But seriously, who knows?

I am continually amazed by the persistence of medical professionals in their quests to measure every aspect of my physical being with precise numbers—and in their attempts to quantify everything into tidy little boxes. When my body and experiences slop and slush over the edges and through the cracks of the cardboard container that I have been assigned, the overflow and the leaks are either randomly quantified in an attempt to neatly tuck them—and me—away, or I am summarily dismissed and ignored.

Ever since returning from the terrible loft incident in Vancouver, I had been struggling for an adequately recognized value in other segments of my life. Suddenly, I had nothing to do but deal with doctors. Blair and I tried to get a line of credit because I couldn't collect my student loan (since I hadn't gone back to school), and I still had flights sitting on my credit card. We met with someone at the bank and explained our situation. She looked us over and said, "Okay, I'll put you down as a homemaker." Laughing in shock, I responded, "That's optimistic on many fronts." But my status as an economic unit had to be quantified to go forward with the application, so I conceded.

We live in a world where it's not enough simply to exist. You have to do something that can be written in the box on your passport. During this period, people would phone me at home in the middle of the day, in the middle of their important lives as productive economic units, and expect me to be perfectly available. So when you have too much time, your time means nothing, has no value, no hourly rate. It shrinks, becoming listless, shrunken, gelatinous, ambiguous, dependant. We internalize the idea that things are of increased value when they are scarce. So we overload our lives with endless activity in order to feel important. The less time we have, the more we can feel that we are of value, that we have a right to exist. At the same time, we are forcibly overloaded by a system that demands that we work more and more for simple survival. Who we *are* is stripped away as we become less and less visible. Wanting to be noticed, not wanting to be seen.

With women, especially, our physical value is determined in a particularly contradictory way. We identify ourselves using numbers that randomly correlate to our physical size and clothing requirements. The phrasing "I'm one-forty" or "I'm an eight," is much more common than "the physical mass of my body weighs one hundred and forty pounds and the number the manufacturer assigns to the clothes required to cover my body is an eight." Our value is at once related to our ability to be strong and competent workers, wives, and mothers and our capacity to maintain the physical appearance of a cardboard cut-out, neatly contained. The Gap now officially has a size zero. So when women are accused of "letting ourselves go" or, more aptly, giving ourselves permission to move away, are we distancing ourselves from being "zero"? Is the frightening cultural element the idea of women having too *much* substance — hollow men frightened of substantive women? In the summer of 2005, I can't help noticing how my massive weight loss, and my subsequent approximation to the size "zero", makes people treat me like a superstar.

9. The First Time We Meet

In the fall, I go to my scheduled appointment with Dr. Loveless, the inflammatory bowel disease specialist.

A doctor I've never seen before enters the examining room. "Hi, I'm Dr. Blackwell. I'm a visiting fellow here doing research with Dr. Loveless, and I'm going to see you today, if that's okay with you."

His accent is from Manchester, the city in England where I was born. I feel warm and safe.

"Yes, that's fine," I say. Then I ask him, "Where are you visiting from?"

"Manchester," he answers. "I'm here with my wife and kids. We're staying for a year."

He's in his thirties, well-spoken, with soft gestures and warm eyes.

"I was born in Manchester," I tell him. "I came here when I was seven."

He lights up, amused and curious. "How long did it take you to get a Canadian accent?"

"Not that long," I say. "But I was already good at faking it before we even moved here."

He shudders. "My daughter just asked me for the stroller the other day." He cringes as he affects a Canadian accent for the word *stroller*.

I laugh heartily at him. "She'll be full-on Canadian by the end of the year."

He asks me to describe what's been going on for me in the last little while. I start describing my symptoms, how I've repeatedly had bowel flare-ups in my internal J-Pouch during the year and four months since the closure surgery. I tell him that I've needed several blood transfusions, because no matter how much iron they inject into me, I'm still severely anemic.

"We'd like to try this new kind of scope on you," he says. "It's a trial, all you need to do is…"

While he's talking and explaining, gently, respectfully, I feel tears welling up in my eyes. My cheeks are getting red and I'm constricting my throat as tightly as I possibly can to suppress the sobs that are threatening to leak out and expose me. Then when I can't hold back any longer, the tears start spilling out of my eyes.

He looks shocked. "What's the matter?"

He's looking around for tissues, and as I reach into my bag and grab my own, he hands me a box and I start wiping my face and explaining. "I just can't. I don't want to have another scope. I've been getting scoped over and over for three and a half years. And the surgeries were supposed to end it. I was supposed to be cured, to feel better. But I'm not and I don't. I feel worse. And they always say scopes don't hurt, but the Fentinel's never enough and they always do hurt. They always do. And I've been so anemic since the surgery that I've had blood transfusions and iron infusions, and I'm so tired and so weak, I've had to delay finishing my master's—I was going to start a PhD this year. And last week I had a stricture stretched out without anaesthetic and I've just had enough. I can't do this anymore."

Enraged, he asks, "Why would they remove a stricture without anaesthetic? Who did that?"

"No, that's not the issue. My surgeon's great. I was already in so much pain from the rectal exam that I agreed she might as well just do it right there instead of booking a room and getting meds. It's not just that. It's everything. It's having to go through this again and again and again."

He's standing very close to me at this point, and rather than looking frightened, disturbed, or annoyed, as I imagined any esteemed bowel specialist would at this point, he's handing me a tissue and saying, "Are you coping?"

It's such a beautiful confluence of events that leads Dr. Blackwell to arrive on the day that I'm suddenly incapable of playing any kind of strategic "patient" role. This is my first and only meltdown at a regular appointment in front of a doctor, much less in the presence of a specialist whom I've only just met. No doctor or nurse in any of the massively traumatic situations I've been in has ever asked me this basic, human question: *Are you coping?* It's so simple, but it alters the dynamic of the encounter so markedly. Suddenly, I'm not just a body on an examining table. Outside of the immediacy of what's happening in my bleeding, leaking body, I'm an entire person whose coping skills are now being held as significant.

I tell him about the work I've been doing with my therapist, Grace. "I've been in a chronic illness support group for the past couple of years. I have emotional support. It's just hard. I'm just getting so fed up."

"I hear this a lot from patients in your situation," he says. "It's so hard after the surgery when things still aren't going as expected, when things are still so difficult. I really think this test could help you, though. Of course, you don't have to do anything you don't want to do, but it's essentially just swallowing a capsule with a camera in it. When we get the images, we can see everything, all the parts, even in the small intestine, that we wouldn't be able to see with a colonoscopy or an endoscope. We might figure out what's causing the anemia. And patients report that this procedure really is painless."

I look up at him and believe him, trust him. He genuinely seems to want to make my life better, not just contain me so he can feel secure that he's managed my disease. So I agree, and he goes out to get Dr. Loveless.

When they return, I'm sitting on the examining table and they're towering over me. Dr. Loveless starts blathering on about what Dr. Blackwell told him and what he wants to do with this information, and as I start looking increasingly shaky again, Dr. Blackwell subtly changes positions so he's standing with me, facing Dr. Loveless from just behind my shoulder, instead of the two of them towering over me. He interjects to answer questions I've already answered. He's shielding me from the cold insensitivity of the standard clinical encounter Dr. Loveless seems intent on acting out. He's a fleecy blanket covering me in the hailstorm of painfully impersonal doctor dialogue.

The procedure goes really well, and the following week, Dr. Blackwell phones me with the results.

"Your results are excellent. Your small bowel looks great. Your pouch is slightly inflamed, but no more than is expected. There's definitely nothing here that would cause your anemia."

Whenever I come in for appointments after this, I see the secretary, Laura, call him from the lab he's working in down the hall. He comes, finds my chart in the stack on her desk, and calls me into the examining room. Clearly, some deal has been brokered. Either Dr. Loveless has assigned him "the difficult patient" or Dr. Blackwell asked specifically for me for his research.

10. Miracles

So I promised we'd get here. It's the final note of my prescription for health care—first money, then manners, then miracles. In a very immediate sense, I feel like I've already described a few. The bottom line for me is that, when it comes down to it, we'll never know how little we know. We can establish general patterns and make general predictions, but ultimately nobody really knows what makes one person with the same genes and the same lifestyle sick and not the other. We don't always know why certain people respond to treatments better than others, and why the same person can be responsive at one time but not at another.

Therefore, I think we always need to be open to other possibilities. The collaboration between my naturopath, GP, and endocrinologist that ultimately cured my adrenal failure is evidence how useful it is to be open-minded. Of course there was science involved, but it was the kind of science that's open to discovery, to the potential that things outside of what we understand can have unforeseen, excellent results. And in this particular situation, none of these practitioners actually spoke to the other. Their teamwork was facilitated by me, and they all trusted me to play this role, to make decisions about who I wanted to work with on what part of my care, and how I wanted this to happen. My anemia leads me to other types of miracles.

So now it's winter, and I'm lying in a hospital bed getting a blood transfusion. No one knows why I still need them, what mystery of anemia and iron deficiency my body is manifesting. Someone has left a New Age spiritual book on the windowsill. Despite the fact that I have my laptop, schoolwork, various novels, political books, and *Buffy* DVDs, I'm feeling an irritating pull toward this book. I feel like I'm being manipulated by the person who left the book sitting there for some vulnerable sick person to find. I picture that person as some kind of hemp-wearing, yogurt-weaving missionary who is overly invested in my enlightenment. I've spent the early part of my twenties carefully cultivating my atheism — partly for reasons of intellectual fashion and partly because I spent my teens fighting with religion teachers in my Catholic school. And yet my desire to read this book just grows. Most likely someone just forgot it there. The chances that it was an intentional plant are pretty slim, but my resistance to it makes me conjure up all kinds of paranoid theories.

It's such a cliché, being sick, feeling like I might die, then finding a brand-new, shiny spiritual freedom with which to save myself. I'm also aware of the narrative cliché that, before any kind of grand spiritual awakening, the protagonist has to demonstrate a respectable level of cynicism. And it's practically an iron-clad rule in memoirs that, before we reveal anything potentially embarrassing that we fear our readers might judge us harshly for, we writers must self-reflexively acknowledge how clichéd we're being.

So sorry, but here I go.

At this point in the story, I've started to meditate really seriously. I'm taking a course and am meditating every day. At first, I found it incredibly challenging, but I've started to enjoy it. Along these lines, I've recently decided that Susie is sending me messages from beyond the grave. Because she was a miniature schnauzer, all of her messengers were little grey furry clones, showing up whenever I needed support or cheering up. I say "decided" rather than "realized" because it just occurred to me at some point that I *liked* believing this. Whether or not it was empirically true, it was making me happy, and that just seemed more important. So that became my new criteria for spiritual belief. *Do I like believing this? Am I hurting anyone?* If the answers were "yes" to the former and "no" to the latter, then a new belief was born. Every time a schnauzer came running up to me, I thanked Susie. I felt a little bit safer in the world, a little more connected, warmer, and protected.

So I pick up the book. And I *like* what the author is saying. I think I would be much happier if I *believed* what she's saying too. Then I realize, much to my surprise, that I do believe it. I believe every word. A month later, I'm lying on a table in a healer's office, talking about spirituality, visions, and meditation. I start seeing this medicine person regularly, talking about all kinds of things in my life and experiencing the effects of hands-on energy healing. The six months after I start seeing her, I am well more often than I'm sick. It's the first time this has been the case in more than six years. She's incredibly supportive about my writing and performing and encourages me to travel and take this work further. Perhaps most importantly, she tells me, "You're strong. Your body is healthy."

This fact is not apparent to anyone else at the time, but as she says it, I feel it to be true. With all my appointments with all of my doctors and specialists, my *health* has been set aside as the entire focus is placed on my *illness*. And there were definitely things about my body that were strong through the whole process. Side effects and symptoms I never had, recoveries from terribly difficult things. I needed someone to acknowledge how incredibly amazing my body was for surviving, for pulling me through to the other side.

But, to be clear, when I suggest "miracles" as a cure for health care, I don't necessarily mean that everyone has to meditate or see energy healers. If people want to, that's great. What I really want to emphasize is that everyone needs to have the option to freely pick and choose the type of care they want, and on their own terms. And all practitioners need to respect this.

II. "Owww!"

It's now February, and my joints are really, really sore. This has happened during bowel flare-ups before, but this time there's no flare-up. They're stiff and inflamed and it's hard to move. This is Tuesday. We have tickets to see Aimee Mann at a club where to see anything you need to stand up near the front. We go, and Blair has to stand behind me to prop me up the whole night.

Thursday morning, I wake up and can barely move at all. Even putting my feet flat on the mattress in front of me hurts my heels and ankle joints too much. I phone Dr. Loveless's office, and Laura, his secretary, tells me that my only option is to go down to emerg. I phone Blair, who's taking a course an hour's drive away. When I explain that I had to slide to the washroom by sitting on a pillow, and it took about twenty minutes, he gets in the car and drives home.

When we get to emerg, someone pages Dr. Blackwell and he comes down to see me. He thinks it might be a virus because it doesn't seem consistent with my colitis. He suggests just taking pain medication until it passes and, if it doesn't improve in a few days, to call him. I'm planning to go to a conference on the weekend, and Adrian and Anna are flying in from Vancouver and staying at our place.

Just before they get in on Friday night, I'm still propped up by lots of cushions and my joints are really bad. I get out *When the Body Says No*, and I look up joint inflammation. I find a section on people with arthritis who don't express their anger or pain—they're completely stoical. I explain this to Adrian and Anna when they arrive. My solution: "So I'm going to be really loud, and really, really complain. Okay?"

I recognize that asking permission to express pain is still pretty dysfunctional, but you know, baby steps.

"Yeah, yeah, yeah, do it! Tell us…" They egg me on.

So I start yelling, at first tentatively, and then enthusiastically. "My joints really fucking hurt! I'm in so much fucking pain. Owww! I fucking hate this!"

Blair joins in. "How much pain?"

"Tons of fucking pain! It's brutal! I'm so pissed off! Owww! This is so unfair!"

We're all laughing, but it feels great.

"So now," I say as I turn to them, "whenever anyone at the conference asks you where I am, you have to say the same thing."

Adrian enthusiastically experiments. "Julie isn't here because her fucking joints hurt! And the pain is fucking unbelievable and it's so unfair!"

We hang out chatting for a while, and then we all go to bed. I sleep through them getting up and leaving in the morning. When I wake up, there is no pain in any of my joints. The inflammation has entirely gone and they don't hurt at all. They're moving with complete ease and flexibility. Blair is amazed. He'd seen the swelling, my inability to move for days. And now it's gone. The following month, I'm sitting in a chair waiting for Dr. Blackwell to come into the examining room. He bounds in energetically and sits up on the examining table. The play of power and space here—him in the traditional place of the patient, me sitting in a chair with a desk next to me—lightens the whole encounter for me. The fearful pit that sits in my stomach before these moments dissolves, and I can focus on what I need to say to him, and how I want to respond, rather than bracing myself for how the doctor might encroach on my body as I occupy the table. He's really shocked that I look so well and I'm so vibrant. I feel vaguely guilty because I clearly got him pretty worried when I came into the emerg.

Then several months later, I go and wait in the hallway near his office while my sister is getting an ultrasound. Joanne's in town for the summer and having some GI pain. She's very healthy and ultimately not diagnosed with anything, but because we share genes, both she and her doctors take any such symptoms very seriously.

Dr. Blackwell walks by and looks shocked to see me.

"Oh, hi. I didn't know you were coming. Do you have an appointment? Are you okay?"

"Yeah, yeah, I'm totally fine. I just came with my sister. She's getting an ultrasound; I'm just waiting."

"Oh, okay."

"I was hoping to catch you before you went back to England."

He's smiling but looking distinctly uncomfortable. "Yeah, I'm still here for another couple of weeks."

"Do you ever give your email to patients?"

"What for?"

At this point, I get slightly irritated, although I'm smiling and genuinely amused at his discomfort. *What for? Oh, I don't know — to discuss nail polish?*

"Um, to talk about my pouch. You always seem to have new ideas and be up on the research, and you answer questions and communicate better than the others."

He looks pleased but says, "No, I don't give it out. You should give the other guys a chance. They're really great; they really know what they're doing. And if you really have a question just for me, then give it to Laura and she'll pass it on to me."

Unlike my surgeon Athena's goddess-secretary, the specialist's secretary, Laura, has always been incredibly rude to me and rarely appears to care enough to demonstrate even the most basic levels of administrative competence. So I look skeptical. "Laura? *Seriously?*"

He laughs loudly and knowingly; clearly he's seen her around the patients.

"Laura's been great. She and I really get along. She'll definitely pass it on."

I guess he's protecting himself from any appearance of impropriety, but it seems pretty extreme to me. I'm hardly going to start sending him naked pictures. He's seen it all anyway. My GP willingly offered me her email address, and the first surgeon I met encouraged me to email him questions so he could send me resources online. I can understand not giving it to *everyone,* but he'd already taken a special interest in my case, and I honestly felt like I was losing a lifeline. An engaged, emotionally competent medical researcher and clinician who was specializing in my disease.

"Well, thanks for everything. Have a good trip home."

He smiles back broadly and looks me right in the eye. "You're welcome."

I do feel a bit lighter as he walks away down the hall. At least I thanked him. In the years to come I practise standing in different ways around the stretcher with med students, experimenting with what works and what doesn't. I find it funny looking back at how Dr. Blackwell just behaved this way naturally, with no artifice—he couldn't possibly have predicted that I would later use him as a case study to model best practices with medical students. Similarly, I wonder if I ended up in any of his research articles as a "problem case."

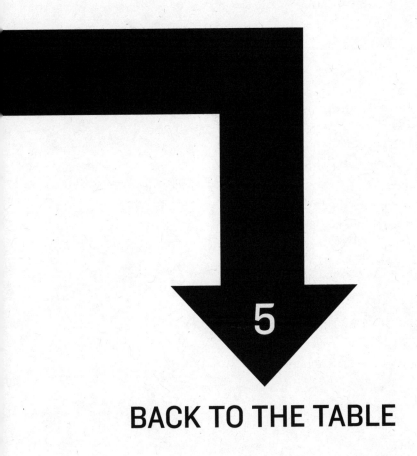

5

BACK TO THE TABLE

I. Leaky Bodies

During my year with Dr. Blackwell, I'm finishing my new master's degree program in Toronto. I'm feeling a growing frustration with the disconnection between my embodied experiences of illness and my academic research.

I'm standing outside the department administrator's office one day when another student approaches. She's wearing a necklace with a Frida Kahlo self-portrait.

"I love Frida!" I practically shout at her.

"*I* love Frida!" she smilingly exclaims back.

"*I* went to her house!" I jokingly brag.

"*I* worked at her house for three months!" she says.

"Okay, you win. I'm Julie, by the way."

"Hi!" She smiles back. "I'm Cristina."

Cristina, who mostly goes by Cris, is an artist and teacher, in school to get her master's degree in the same area as I am. We almost immediately start plotting how we can collaborate on a project using Frida Kahlo's art. We ultimately discover an opportunity in our methodology course and put together a project by pouring through paintings of hers, some of which Cris knows and I've never even seen before. One of these is called *Without*

Hope. Frida is lying in bed, against the barren backdrop with solar-system planets spinning above, with what she describes as the "jaws of life" in her mouth. But in these jaws of life, there's human viscera, skulls, fish heads, and animals. According to Cris, Frida described this painting as depicting her frustration with the medical establishment, with years of having things shoved down her throat.

I learn from these paintings in a way and with a depth and intensity that's hard to articulate. Frida teaches me that you can't fake art using some formulaic method you learned in grad school. Everyone's seen some form of educational theatre or after-school special type of cringe-worthy, committee-approved endeavour. It's always highly mockable. The annoying thing about creating art is that it needs to be more spontaneous and more laborious than that. Picking off the scab and poking through the wound, feeling through the pain to magically transport ourselves (and hopefully our audience) to some place different. The most valuable, incredible information can sit on shelves and gather dust. When art comes from a genuine, terrifying place, it keeps theories, ideas, and research alive.

The raw and bloody writing in my hospital notebooks keeps floating to the forefront of my consciousness. So when we hold a student conference, I produce a large backdrop based on *Without Hope*, with a reproduction of the painting in the centre. I take my writing about my illness and create pages with parallel columns—on the left is my writing about illness, on the right brilliant and beautiful academic quotes about illness. I'm discovering theories and theorists who speak about bodies and illness in a way that I can actually relate to.

One such theorist, Margrit Shildrick, is at the conference. She writes about "leaky bodies," a feminist concept that explains how women's bodies don't "fit" into the constructs of bodies set up by modern Western philosophies. So in the early years of medical science, male bodies were studied as the "norm"—even medications intended for women were tested on men because science couldn't control or account for the cyclical unpredictability of women's menstruating bodies. How, then, could medical professionals relate to these messy, leaky, out-of-control women?

Margrit is visiting from Ireland as an adjunct professor to our faculty, and I'm really excited to meet her. She gives me warm and kind feedback on my presentation, and I ask to meet her in the coming days.

She agrees, but when I actually arrive at her office and ask her to supervise me, she says, "I'm going back to Ireland, I really won't be available to supervise students here."

I smile and respond with complete honesty, "I really don't like being supervised, and I'm really low maintenance."

She smiles back. "Well, it is possible, but it's just nice being in the same place. We could talk on the phone, but it's not the same as being able to meet in person and having a cup of tea."

"Yeah, I do understand, but I'd really like to work with you, and I really am pretty independent."

So Margrit agrees to supervise me, and I'm thrilled. My department puts my poster presentation up in a glass display case. I'm pleased that they like it that much, but a bit horrified that it's the first thing people see when they get off the elevator. I run into the director of my program one day, right in front of the glass case, and she tells me how many positive comments she's had about it. I just feel so exposed. I tell her, "I feel like I'm literally leaking off the cardboard page with my colon poetry."

She laughs, which in retrospect I can understand; it is a bit of dramatic thing to hear when you're not expecting it. But it's exactly how I'm feeling.

I inwardly cringe with embarrassment and cheerfully say, "That's what it's all about right? Our leaking bodies..."

Very quietly, without really telling anyone what I'm about to do, I apply to a couple of large conferences in my field, with my new idea of a "performance piece." The idea that occurred to me in that bed-blocking lecture crystallizes and solidifies while I spend the better part of the following year stuck in my apartment, unable to take classes. On a certain level, I see this performance as separate from my studies, an "un-academic" departure. It's a cheeky idea that makes me smile because I just can't see myself giving *papers* about chronic illness sitting behind tables anymore. But much to my surprise, and if I'm honest, my initial horror, all the conferences invite me to come and perform.

And when I tell Margrit what I've been doing, I half expect her to be annoyed that I've taken such a departure from thesis reading and work. She's briefly in town again, so we are actually meeting over cups of tea. Instead of disapproving, as I'd feared she might, she insists that this performance work be central to my master's research and encourages me to integrate audience reactions into my research. So I organize my proposal based on all of the stories I wrote while I was sick.

There are four sections: The Stretcher, The Table, The Theatre, and The Recovery Room. I begin each conference piece by taking my clothes off and putting on a hospital gown. I sit on a makeshift stretcher, created from an academic table and a hospital sheet, and start reading from what looks like a metal chart.

The first time I do it is at a conference in Toronto, in front of lots of people I know. Beforehand, Blair and I are sitting on a bench outside when it suddenly hits me how badly this could potentially go. "Is this a really, really bad idea?" I ask him, "What's wrong with me?"

He laughs. "No, it's a really great idea, it's going to be super-good."

"But I'm not an actor, I've barely even practised. How am I going to do the voices?"

And then Blair miraculously comes up with a brilliant idea that gets me through. "Every time you play a nurse, imitate your dad imitating your mum. For doctors, do your mum imitating your dad."

He's referring to my family's habitual dinner practice of bickering about the days' events in a very dramatic he-said-she-said format.

So I try it. "Like this? *Memememimahama.*" I say it in a high pitch. "And, *Mumreumerumemuh.*" This time I use an improbably low caveman-esque voice.

"Exactly!"

Blair and I are both laughing on the bench now, and I feel lighter, ready to perform.

And so My Leaky Body, the project, is born. Here I begin Stretcher Journey Number Two, the redux. From a bed-blocker in emergency wards to a basket case in post-surgical recovery, to a performer of the socio-politics of the Canadian health care system, talking about the cultural implications of being a young woman with a chronic illness. Wearing a hospital gown at the *front* of the room, occupying the place of a knowledgeable teacher. I use a PowerPoint presentation. Partially for irony and partially to give people Frida paintings and academic quotes to situate my story in something bigger than me. And, if I'm honest, to give people somewhere to look, other than just at me. Because of the potential trauma of this idea, I have a little inside joke with myself when I design the slides. I use a font called Impact, which I always think of as an activist font, reserved for bold political posters calling people to action. Every time I see the overhead screen out of the corner of my eye with academic words in commie font, I smile quietly to myself and continue performing.

I continually worry about being self-indulgent—that my story is too personal and the content too gross. All my fears wash away as people react during and after the performances. The most unexpected people connect to my story and support me in finding new venues. And the more I perform in these different places, the more I'm aware of how much performing I was doing all along, through my illness, through endless hospitalizations, through months of being in bed and on the toilet. In each moment, as my body spun out of control, I asked myself, *Which character am I going to play right now?* The stoic young woman, the emotional patient, the good student, the loving friend? It's not that there was no truth in any of these roles, they just weren't always a reflection of how I genuinely felt in those moments. And here, bringing all of these roles into performance, exposing my raw wounds to people who relate and connect and understand, is freeing me somehow. I start to see, and really believe, that, out of all of this horror and pain, something good, something exciting, some kind of adventure is emerging. Clouds only have silver linings when you paint them on—and now I finally have my opportunity to slather shiny, gilded edges onto the black storm clouds of the past five years.

2. Ashes & Crows

A year later, I'm performing all over the place and getting media attention. I get my first paid conference booking that I have to travel to. It's for the Disability Health Research Network (DHRN) in Vancouver. Valorie Crooks, one of my professors and thesis committee members from my master's, is on their board and recommends that they bring me out for their event. It's the first time I've been back to Vancouver since my adrenal meltdown almost four years earlier. As I'm packing to leave, I look up at the little shelf where I keep Susie's ashes. In all of my multiple hospitalizations in the months and years surrounding her death, people brought me little stuffed schnauzers, so by now I have a pile of Susie look-alikes. They surround her urn, with one on top wearing her collar. On an impulse, I wrap the urn and take it with me.

When I arrive in Vancouver, it feels like a completely different city. Adrian picks me up from the airport, and we go back to his and his partner Anna's apartment. I remember how one of the first times I hung out with Anna was in Toronto during the summer following my disastrous attempt to return. She and Adrian and Blair and I are sitting in my parents' backyard. I'm recovering from surgery.

"Julie," she says, "the next time you almost die in an apartment by yourself, can you *not* wait until 7:00 a.m. to phone someone? Maybe just call right away."

I laugh, explaining that part of the problem was I was so out of it I wasn't thinking straight. She continues to look sternly at me until I agree. "Okay, next time I almost die, I'll phone someone right away."

She smiles. "Thanks."

Now in Vancouver, in much calmer circumstances, Adrian and I are sitting in their apartment having tea and lunch before he drives me to the hotel where I'm staying. When I get up to the room the DHRN has booked for me, I almost fall over. It's beautiful: huge, bright, wide-open. Gorgeous view and stylish patterns.

I have fun at the event and meet lots of lovely people. That night, my former professor Valorie takes me and another guest speaker out to a fancy fish restaurant in Stanley Park. This is Vancouver as I've never experienced it—and it's glorious. The following morning, I pack Susie's ashes into my backpack and take the bus to our old neighbourhood. I walk around and down to the beach where Susie was last playful and happy. I reach a small cove and sit down. A crow perches on a rock about arm's length from me. I decide there and then to release little Susie. I do a small ceremony befitting my dog, as the crow sits very still, looking on. When I walk away from the beach, about a hundred crows that I couldn't see from my cove suddenly take flight. They'd been perched on wires and in trees and they all flap away, their wings beating in rhythm with the ocean waves. I watch them as they fly out of view. Vancouver used to be a dark, grey place, where wintertime meant several hours of a slightly brighter grey sky around noon before another night of seemingly interminable darkness. It's now a place of magical crows, beautiful spaces, and warm, kind people.

3. Because Bums Are Funny

A short time later, I finally get my first request to do interactive workshops with health care professionals. I've been offering and fantasizing about doing these kinds of workshops for a while, but this is the first time someone actually takes me up on it. It's for a large conference in Alberta. They ask me to do a performance to the hundreds of doctors, nurses, and front-line managers in their plenary, and then run break-out workshops in the afternoon with groups of forty. I accept the booking a year in advance thinking I have lots of time to come up with something good to do in the afternoon.

As the time approaches, I'm performing in a theatre festival in Toronto and totally consumed with the effort. The month before the event I rack my brain about which scene from my life to turn into an educational exercise. I decide somewhat impulsively that I'd love for health care professionals to *feel* (or at least imagine that they're feeling) what it's like to get something as routine as a rectal exam while consumed by the pain of a chronic bowel disease.

When I wake up in my hotel room the morning of the conference, I panic. I've prepared a PowerPoint presentation to accompany the exercise and I have notes and a sequence of events that seems reasonable to play out in the timeline. But until this moment, it doesn't actually occur to me that I've planned to re-enact a mock rectal exam based on one of the most traumatic moments in my experience, with large groups of health care professionals who I've never met before. And I panic. Now, my version of panic is rarely discernible to the naked eye. It usually involves me sitting very still and being very quiet. Inside, I'm quivering and screaming, but outside I look calm. I still have several hours before I perform, so I go through a list of options. I could hide under the bed. I could hide under the quilt on the bed. I could take a really deep bath and hide underwater. Or I could get out of the hotel room. Wisely, I choose the last option. I get into my rental car and drive to the nearest coffee shop. I sit with my laptop, reviewing my notes, and realizing that this is all I have prepared, so I'm just going to have to go for it.

When I return to the hotel for the conference, people are incredibly nice. For possibly the first time ever, doing the actual show feels easy and almost soothing. At least, I know what's going to happen. The audience is warm and enthusiastic in their responses. And then, the workshops. So I'm standing in front of a group of forty health care professionals who've signed up to learn better communication skills. I'm holding a gown and a glove. I ask for two volunteers. The description in their program advertised mock clinical interactions, but now that they've seen the content of my show, they look unsure.

"I promise that no actual rectal exams will be performed."

Everyone starts laughing and two people get up.

I make the offer. "Gown or glove?"

They choose, and we all watch while the one with the gown awkwardly struggles to put it on. This is part of the point. I ask the one wearing the gown to read the description I wrote six years earlier for Dr. Singer, and I ask the crowd to concentrate on the instructions:

So here's an exercise. Put your hand on the very front of your collarbone. The two bumps in the centre of your chest at the base of your throat. Imagine someone has tied a string around the passageways directly above and behind this bone. Those you use for eating, drinking, breathing. The strings are attached to strings coming from the back of your nasal cavities and throat and are being pulled down into your gut. Your rectum and the area just on the inside of each hip feel sore, aching, and expanded, like a weight. The strings have pulled these areas up and have become tangled. Every time you move, you are at risk of retching and spasming. All of these movements are caught up with one another. You are weak, tired, shaky, and dizzy.

As I look around the room, I'm amazed. Everyone is very carefully concentrating and following my instructions. When we get to the scenario where I direct them in acting out what happened between Dr. Singer and me, they giggle at the awkwardness of imitating this violating experience between two colleagues and gasp at the horror of what happened to me. When we follow up with discussion and redo the scene to make it more ethical and respectful, people express how much more comfortable *everyone* is in the second scenario — the person performing the mock rectal exam as well as the one receiving it.

The actual intimacy of this and other procedures is constantly denied in one manner or another. And yet, as I engage health care professionals and students in my mock rectal exam exercises, we inevitably all end up laughing. Bums are funny. The suggestion that one of my volunteers will pretend to penetrate another's bum with their gloved hand is funny. It suggests sexual play and a public crossing of boundaries. A shared violation of cultural taboos. It does not make anyone less competent or trustworthy as a health care provider to acknowledge this. Certainly, I don't want anyone giggling when they actually perform a procedure on me. But the complete denial of the very obvious human intimacy involved promotes coldness and insensitivity on the part of the provider. And this detachment clearly contributes to situations that have caused trauma for me.

We follow up with a storytelling exercise where the participants give their impressions and tells their own stories from their own experiences. We discuss what works and what doesn't, moments where they've felt supported in their practice, and moments that have ended badly. The thing I hear most often now that I've been doing these types of workshops more regularly is, "Why don't we get to do this more often?"

Some have suggested implementing these types of discussions as a regular feature in the clinics and hospitals where they work. For me, it's important that we sit with the fact that we don't have clear answers for "what to do" and "how to fix" things.

"We are still at the beginning of this conversation," I tell them, "with patients coming forward more than ever before, and demanding to be included in discussions of health care delivery. So let's have this conversation. Let's look at what works and what doesn't — not to judge it, or to blame individuals. Not to come up with quick-fix answers. Just to observe and record based on our actual experiences and see what comes out of that."

In a nursing class, one of the students asks me, "Are you ever going to make this a real play?"

I'm puzzled by the question, so I ask what she means.

"You know, like with other people playing the other parts."

The whole point is that this is just my perspective, my story. I'm not claiming that I'm faithfully recounting word for word with eerily accurate impressions that this is what happened. I'm saying that from my perspective, flat on my back, this is how I experienced it. Of course, my heightened emotions of terror and mistrust colour my memories. But I don't think my emotional realities could possibly be that divorced from the experiences of vast numbers of patients, so it may have some educational value for health practitioners. In the same vein, I also think that when professionals discuss a patient, make a declaration, or write something in their chart for other professionals to read and make judgments on, that's just their perspective, their story.

Over the years of doing this work, I get to fulfill the fantasy that got me through being a medical education project and teaching tool—I finally get to teach manners to med students.

4. Manners for Med Students

"Actually, I was in on a scope yesterday where the woman kept asking them to stop and they wouldn't. She was in a lot of pain, and no matter how much medication they gave her, it still hurt. But because she had consented before the procedure and now she was *high*, we didn't stop." The med student is standing in front of her whole class, her voice shaking. "It was painful to watch," she tells us.

I've just taught rounds at their hospital—stripping at the front of the room and awkwardly struggling with my gown while they pretend not to squirm. Performing scenes from my stretcher and getting volunteers to re-enact my most traumatic rectal exam. A student in the audience has just claimed, "We would never do that, that's not proper protocol." And this brave student responds to her colleague by describing her experience in a real-life procedure the day before. In our exercise, she was just lying on the stretcher, essentially playing me. She still has my gown on while she's talking. The student who is playing doctor is still wearing his rectal-ready latex glove. "Well, yes," he counters. "They need their secum statistics."

I ask what he means.

"Well, the secum is the area at the end of the colon attaching..." He's gesturing an outline of the colon for me indicating that the secum is where the large intestine connects to the small one.

"Right, but what's the statistic?"

"Doctors need to keep their statistics for reaching the secum high to keep their funding—that's what is considered a successful scope."

And I'm totally horrified. I had no idea. I can immediately see the medical rationale here. The idea of a colonoscopy is to obtain images and tissue samples for biopsy. The more of the colon that is seen and biopsied, the more early detections of cancer and other bowel diseases are possible. So a doctor who is consistently able to scope entire colons is considered successful and will be funded to perform these procedures.

Fast-forward to the patient—that embodiment of disease, that bearer of a colon. Lying on the table, the patient's attitude and body become barriers to a physician's success. These barriers can be overcome by sedating the fight out of us and, ultimately, by the fact that patients are lying prone and almost naked, while physicians are supported by a team of awake, alert, and strong bodies who are fully clothed, then draped and masked. The limitations of a success-failure model in patient care are clear in this scenario. Clinical success is directly proportional to bodily violation. Conversely, clinical failure results from listening to and respecting the patient's expressions.

As we wrap up these scenes in these "safe" workshop moments, I'm always warmed to see how medical students and health care professionals bring their full selves to the table. Often they improvise. One particularly funny student makes a great display of waving his gloved finger like an evil scientist while the rest of his classmates cringe. I surprise myself by finding this genuinely amusing. We move quickly out of the first scenario into a second scenario that I've developed based on my deepest desires of what a scope experience *could* look like. Every single time, every single person in the room expresses how relieved, comfortable, and safe they feel in the second scenario. And the person who always expresses this the most emphatically is the one wearing the glove. As one male medical student puts it, referring to his female colleague playing patient, "I just felt so much better about it when she was saying what she wanted and I listened to her. The first time I felt really scared."

And this is from a scenario where no one even touched anyone. I can't imagine the intensity of the feeling he would be having if he actually penetrated her anus with his gloved finger. And yet, in most clinical interactions, this honest acknowledgement of feeling is strictly verboten. The thing that always stands out for me the most is how ill-equipped health care professionals feel when dealing with emotional trauma—their own and their patients'. So much of a clinical interaction is shaped by and shrouded in huge, unspoken emotions.

In the follow-up discussion, I give an anecdote from the previous week, where my GP walks into the examination room and tells me how exhausted she is and what time she has been working since. I think about all the health care professionals who have said at other workshops that their colleagues should not be "dumping" their own emotional realities onto patients whose situations are so much worse than their own.

I disagree with this objection for two reasons. The first reason is that I am already pretty sensitive. If someone is having any kind of issue when they approach me, often I already know, so I feel more comfortable if they acknowledge it. In my experience, those physicians and nurses who fail to acknowledge their own situations in an honest way are more likely to take their bad mood out on me in an indirect way.

The second reason is that I think the emphasis for health care professionals to set aside their own personal experiences of caregiving in order to provide services is fundamentally problematic, both for the patient and for the professional. For the patient, it suggests that we truly are the "broken" ones, and that the only people capable of "fixing" us must be perfect and flawless. As long as the facade of feeling nothing and maintaining a cool and problem-free exterior is the mainstay of professional conduct, the patient gets established as the imperfect, messy problem. The upshot for me is that clinical encounters tend to be more effective when I feel some modicum of equality with the clinician. I find any acknowledgment of imperfection comforting rather than burdensome.

And this tension is reflected in how intensely medical students look for immediate, concrete solutions to everything we discuss: from dilemmas I raise to their own problems and ones that their classmates share. Students become frustrated when they can't provide one. I tell them about the year I was seeing Dr. Blackwell. We didn't *solve* anything, but I felt the clinical interactions really "worked" because I was being listened to and learning things. For me, as a patient, it's incredibly important to feel like an active participant in my own care.

One student has been looking pretty skeptical in moments throughout the entire workshop. She pipes up, "But some patients are just such poor historians. They come in with these vague descriptions of symptoms. Just saying 'It hurts' and pointing at locations that could be anywhere. You don't know what medication they've taken or when they last saw a health care professional."

I agree that this can be frustrating, and as we continue talking, she suddenly comes out with something that I totally don't see coming. "And last week we had a patient who came in, and by the time I got in to see him, he was dead. We couldn't revive him. The waiting room was packed, so I just had to go straight out and see other patients."

She looks shaken. I can just picture her parting the curtains on the stall, going from someone who just died, straight into a big shift with a million demands from people who've been waiting.

"How awful," I say. "What did you need to happen?"

A classmate answers for her. "At the very least, ten minutes alone just to catch a breath in-between!"

The first woman nods. "Yes, that would've helped."

I can't see how training these amazing young people to ignore the depth of life-and-death situations and the gravity of their own reactions is ultimately helpful to patients. No wonder she gets frustrated when her next patient comes in with ailments she can't pinpoint or understand. She needed someone to talk to, some space to process the fact that something huge just happened. By her own reckoning, when she doesn't get that, she has even less compassion to offer her next patient.

5. She Gives Good Scope

My life unfolds like a spiral—I continually revisit the same areas but from a slightly different position. Less than five percent of patients who are diagnosed and go through treatment and surgery for ulcerative colitis ultimately have their diagnosis changed to Crohn's disease. And, dum-dada-dum, I am one of that elite group.

It starts with an appointment with my GP in the fall of 2008. I've mostly been great for the past couple of years. Taking care of my health is still a priority, but it's not the only thing I do anymore. I've been travelling and performing, actually making a living providing health care workshops. My GP discovers what she refers to as an "ano-rectal fistula at six o'clock," which to me sounds kind of like a cocktail. It turns out that it's just an ulcer, but when she gets the letter from my GP, Athena wants to scope me anyway.

It's the first scope I've had in years, the only one I've ever had done by Athena herself. She's amazing. She waits until the meds are working and goes in so gradually it doesn't hurt at all. She talks to me the whole time. There's a stricture, where my rectum becomes really narrow, at the site where my J-Pouch was attached to my rectum. The scar tissue is practically blocking it shut. In addition, there's a small tunnel, a fistula, between this area and my vagina. This entire area looks quite diseased on the scope.

It's hard to explain how this information kind of feels like good news. I still have issues with rectal bleeding and pain, and although I try to limit my use of antibiotics, I do end up feeling they're necessary more often than I would like. After seeing the extent of the infected ulcerations, Athena immediately gives me a prescription for antibiotics. And at this time, the pain and discomfort for me isn't even the worst its been. It's somehow validating that she's taking it so seriously. When she sees me in her office a week later she doesn't meet my eyes in the waiting room. She hates giving me bad news. Sometimes, I wonder whether I remind her of someone specifically—a sister, a close friend—or if she's like this with all her patients. I mean I'm sure she's great with everyone; I just can't imagine being able to sustain the intensity of her very genuine compassion and carry a surgical practice. She tells me that she feels pretty certain my diagnosis actually is Crohn's disease.

I spend a couple of days feeling really scared of the new diagnosis. And then it just kind of hits me it's what I've already had all this time—and I'm doing just fine. Diagnoses, prognoses, they're just a collection of facts about other people's bodies; they're not crystal balls. They're useful information, not absolute decrees. If I have Crohn's disease, I've had it for seven years now, and I'm feeling all right. I've learned how to take care of myself. A diagnosis is just an explanation for something that already is. I'm living in this body. I know what it does and what's it's like and how it feels. A different set of words doesn't change that.

Since Dr. Blackwell left, I've been avoiding seeing Dr. Loveless, my original gastroenterologist.

Athena gives me the surgical options I may need at some point, and she wants me to talk to someone to see if there are other medication options with my new diagnosis. I ask if she can get me Dr. Gold, the really warm and kind man who met me in the emerg three weeks before our wedding.

In our first appointment, he's really great. He's receptive to what I'm telling him and gives me lots of information. He's genuinely interested in my work and suggests that he'd love to come to a workshop because he might learn something. And then he says he'd like to scope me himself and try manually stretching out the stricture.

I begin the day of the scope on my bathroom floor attempting to give myself a warm-water enema. As I lie prone on the bath mat, I tell myself that it's like having a warm bath inside. Which, although quite convincing to my brain, is less convincing to my strictured rectum. Blair comes home from work, and we head to the hospital. We're very nonchalant about these types of routines these days. The scope unit has been completely redone and it's extremely shiny and fancy looking now. There are bathrobes for patients to accompany our gowns, but still no slippers. The change rooms are pretty, and buoyed by my recent and fabulous scope experience with Athena, I'm feeling good.

The porter who comes to collect me is a super-nice guy, comforting and funny all at once. The nurses are chatty, friendly, and respectful. And then it all goes downhill. The meanest, most abrupt nurse appears out of nowhere to assist Dr. Gold in my scope. And as soon as he has a hose in his hand, Dr. Gold suddenly transforms into cold, businesslike doctor-man.

The nurse starts my meds and Dr. Gold immediately has his gloved hand up my ass.

"Wait!" I say. I wince, sucking in my breath and reflexing away from him. "The meds aren't working yet."

He lets out an exasperated sigh and says, "I'm just putting cream on!"

Considering he's seen my ulcerated anus during our office visit, I can't understand what's confusing him here. He continues putting his finger up inside of me and starts stretching out my narrowed rectum.

"Owww!" I yell.

He ignores me, so I scream.

He pulls his finger out and says angrily, "Don't scream again!"

I start crying.

"Shhh!" he instructs sharply. "Don't cry!"

He motions to the nurse. "Get some wet cloths and wipe her face."

As if my tears are some kind of open wound in need of a tourniquet. *If the fluid leaking from the patient's eyes can be adequately absorbed by the towels, then the problem will be solved.*

This is the first time I have ever cried during a physical exam or scope. The fact that I did this time speaks not just to the extreme pain and physical trauma, but also to my brand-new emotional health and competence. I can tell that he thinks I'm a hysteric and has completely dismissed me as a credible source of any information. The truth is, in this moment, I am more real, more present, and in my opinion, more credible than ever before.

And I'm not just crying because he hurt me. Though the pain and shock certainly triggered the tears. I'm crying because I can't believe this is happening. I've just spent the past two months educating hundreds and hundreds of health care professionals about appropriate ways to communicate with patients. The mock rectal exams we did worked partially because bums are funny and partially because everyone was horrified about the concept of violating someone's ass without getting *real* consent.

I'm still crying on the gurney in the recovery area, tears of exhaustion as much as anything else. I'm so mind-blowingly tired of fighting. I sit up and start to get dressed. Dr. Gold comes to see me. "You need to lie down. You've had a lot of medication."

I look up at him. "I feel totally fine."

He turns to one of the nice nurses I met earlier. "Pull her curtain closed and turn that light out so she sleeps." As if I'm a three-year-old refusing to nap. He walks away.

The nurse looks in and sees that I'm crying. "Oh no," she says. "You should never leave here feeling bad, or like you've done anything wrong. You have not done anything wrong. I know it's easy for me to say, but this is not personal."

So we're at *this* moment again. I know it well. An incredible, brave, strong, angelic nurse descends from the heavens (okay, more likely rushes in from another crisis, which I guess makes it more impressive) to vindicate all my feelings of horror about a physician's behaviour. From this vantage point, the nurse always appears to me to be bestowed with a magical sort of beauty. She does not apologize for him. In fact, she often gives me accounts of his history of temper tantrums. Usually, she indicates in some way that it's not personal. By which I believe she means it's not my fault. Which is great. For whatever dysfunctional reason, in that moment, I need to hear that none of this is my fault. But not *personal*?

My pain is personal. Violations of my body are personal. My flashbacks of every traumatic rectal examination or scope I've ever received are personal. My screams, my tears, my trembling body are all of my person. They are personal.

In the evening, I go to my yoga class. The one tonight is mostly meditation, so I figure it'll be okay. I tell my teacher that I've just come from a medical procedure that afternoon, so I'll be taking things very slowly.

She looks at me and says, "You're very brave."

My initial reaction to such remarks is always a slight discomfort. I always feel like a bit of a fraud, and part of me wants to say, "Well, it wasn't really a big deal, it wasn't that bad." Or, "That's not why I'm telling you…" I'd hate anyone to think I'm looking for such a response.

But, today, I just nod acknowledgment and take my place on the floor.

When I lie in bed at night, I think of all the things I'm grateful for. To be clear, I don't do this because of some moralistic sense that I *should* be grateful. I do it because I've learned that I can choose to like my life, and then I feel happier. And I like that. I also need my expressions of gratitude to the universe to be absolutely true, or it doesn't work. So I start small. "I am grateful that dude's finger is not up my ass right now." That's true. "I'm grateful that I know how painful it is to have dude's finger up my ass because I remember how awesome it is to *not* be in pain." Which is potentially unconvincing to people who haven't had years of debilitating pain in their lives, but for me, it works. "I'm grateful that I don't have to do that again for a long, long time." Definitely, indisputably true. So that's the hard part done. Being thankful for all the lovely things comes easily. And then I fall asleep.

I wake up again in the middle of the night and suddenly feel the need to write my day. This hasn't happened for a really long time, and I've been secretly wondering if I'll *ever* want to write about this type of material again or get back to my old manuscript to turn it into a book. I realize that I am grateful for the experience with Dr. Gold for one more reason—finally, finally, finally, I can't stop writing. I take myself back hours into the day into the pain and horror, and I see that in this moment, as he retreats from his digital assault, he pulls the plug on my writer's block. If this moment were animated, the last frame would be the doctor, looming above me, inspecting his giant finger, while beautiful fairy-like wild flowers burst from my ass in an elaborate bouquet. Glorious.

6. But We Tried to Help You

When she approaches me in the parking lot, I have that little conversation in my head that I always find myself having in situations like this. *Should I be nervous? I'm not nervous, but she totally attacked me in there. What do I do?*

So I smile warmly and say, "Hi."

Her eyes are still a bit red and puffy. She smiles back tentatively. "I'm sorry for being so negative in there."

"You have nothing to apologize for. I'm so glad you brought up politics." I lean in and say quietly, "I wasn't allowed to, which is pretty ridiculous when you think about it."

She looks uncomfortable. Perhaps she doesn't see her remarks about her working conditions as "political."

She jiggles her car keys, ready to walk away, and then says, "I just want to thank you. I've really been thinking about what you said. Especially what you said about the young med students. Because you're right. They're trail-blazing, and you, you're a trailblazer too."

It's four months after my re-diagnosis and painful scope with Dr. Gold. I'm doing a provincial tour for a western health network. The parking lot scene happens after the first engagement on the tour, a performance in a long-term care facility.

A couple of hours earlier, the scene goes like this: I walk up to the front of the room silently, lift up a wrinkled hospital gown that is draped across a chair, and lay it out on the stretcher. I slowly start peeling off my dress, my boots, my socks. Then I change into my gown and walk toward the audience. With the snap of my latex glove, it all begins.

The network has sent an ethicist to co-facilitate the discussions after my performances. The ethicist, who is called Michelle, faces me while I'm performing and doesn't see all the puffy, tear-filled eyes behind her as I tell my story. The organizers asked me to focus on the theme of "transitions" for health care workers, so I decide to talk about my own physical transition from Human to Ostomate. It's the first time I've performed the contents of the "Reformed" chapter, and I'm surprised to find how intensely everyone is reacting. I talk about everything from the Cheshire Cat Resident to Dinah, the home care nurse, who supported me in feeling functional again.

My presentation is based on the concept that everyone working in a health care facility is constantly supporting people in moving through transitions. Starting with birth, through surgeries and other medical interventions, to the final transition from life to death, health care workers become expert at confronting transitional stages. Many health care professionals have amazing skills in getting people through these times, but how often do they apply these skills to take care of themselves? The provincial government has recently fired all the heads of the health regions within the province and is amalgamating those regions. Nobody knows what the new health care structure will look like, whether they'll keep their job, and if they do, how much their working conditions will deteriorate. *This* is what is now being branded as a "transition." I have a long-standing fantasy that I am part of a picket line outside a hospital (wearing my gown, of course), carrying a sign that reads "Their working conditions are my healing conditions."

In many circumstances, I heartily believe in framing things in a positive way. So rather than arguing that we're all screwed, health care is being destroyed, and there's nothing you can do, I point out that the only way we got our public health care system, which in its heyday was the envy of the world, was through the collaboration and cooperation of masses of people, starting at their kitchen tables and ending in the streets and in the legislatures—and we can do that again. To me, the framing of an intentional destruction of the health care system by governments who favour private insurance as simply a "transition" that we can all embrace seems a lot more like dangerous denial than like empowering positivity. But the organizers explicitly asked me not to be political, openly saying that it could affect their funding. Which already seemed a bit odd to me, because the woman I had this conversation with is fantastically smart and educated, bright and funny and grounded, and she had *seen* the show—Tommy Douglas descending from the heavens and all.

But I agreed, and so here I am. I'm telling all the rough and bloody details, without any mention of staff working conditions, overcrowding, funding cuts, or the uplifting idea that Tommy Douglas will save us and that a beautiful new health care system can be dreamed into fruition under anaesthetic. And people look miserable. Some are openly crying; many are staring straight ahead, just looking exhausted and fed up. I wrap up the performance. People clap, and the hospital social worker who organized this particular event thanks me and presents me with a giant bouquet of long-stemmed pink roses. No one's ever given me flowers at this kind of event before. Classy.

While Michelle, the ethicist, gets up to introduce the workshop segment, a number of the people in the room get up to go. I interject, "Please don't leave. This is the part that will cheer you up." Some participants have work shifts starting soon but agree to stay until the last possible moment. We break into small groups so they have a chance to talk through some of the issues that came up in the performance in a more secure way than out loud in front of everyone. When we open up the discussion, people spend a lot of time apologizing to me about things in my story that they feel shouldn't have happened to me.

"Thank you, I really appreciate you saying that," I tell them. "But I do get how these situations happen, and for me, the point is for us to talk about ways to support everyone in these moments. Not to blame. So you really don't need to feel bad. I don't believe health care professionals wake up in the morning wanting these things to happen, and I don't think this is what anyone is anticipating when they choose to be a nurse, a doctor, a technologist." Someone sniffles loudly. Lots of people nod.

Michelle is really interested in discussing all the ethics violations in the health care scenes of my performance in-depth, and starts naming them and asking people to explore what was wrong with what was done to me. This is definitely not lifting the mood of the crowd.

I click through PowerPoint slides, skipping ahead to steer the discussion toward remembering moments in their careers when stressful things occurred where they felt supported by their co-workers—and remembering what this looked like. People break into small groups to discuss this. I lean in to speak quietly to Michelle at the front of the room. "People were really emotionally stimulated during the performance."

She looks at me kind of indifferently and shrugs. "Yeah..."

"No, I mean, like, they were crying. People got really upset."

She looks so surprised that I start to wonder if I imagined it. Then I look back at the still puffy eyes of the participants and tell her, "So I really want to focus on possibilities for positive change."

We gather the group back together, and people start sharing their stories. One woman is getting increasingly impatient at the back of the room. She's wearing hospital scrubs, has her blond curly hair tied back, her eye makeup is smudged, and her nose is very red. She puts her hand up, and I acknowledge her and welcome her to speak. She says, "Hi, I'm Laurie, and I just want to play devil's advocate for a minute."

Her tone is so hostile that I remind myself to take a deep breath as I wait for what comes next.

"How do medical students and doctors react when you perform this?"

The actual content of her question is so mild that I know she must actually want to say something else, something much harsher, but I answer.

"On the whole, really positively. Much better than I initially anticipated when I started doing these performances. Professionals tend to see themselves and their own experiences reflected..."

She explodes, interrupting me. "But people *tried* to help you! We did everything we could and you just kept saying 'no,' so what could we do? When I have twelve patients who need me and I'm offering things and people aren't accepting what I'm offering what am I supposed to *do?*"

I immediately start to feel defensive, and a cheeky little part of me wants to put on my best psychotherapist voice and say, *Are you feeling angry with me right now? Because that's okay*...But before I even get a chance to answer, about five people in the audience respond with remarks like, "She's only human!" and "She was scared!" and "People aren't always ready to receive help at the exact moment we're ready to offer it!"

And I say, "I purposely tell parts of the story where I'm not perfect. I'm telling the truth. The point isn't that I'm an ideal patient, it's that we're all humans in really difficult and traumatic situations that are highly wrought with emotion. Patients shouldn't have to be perfectly well behaved in order to be treated with respect. And we need to collaborate on ways to make these moments work better for *everyone*."

Laurie slumps farther back into her chair, sort of muttering, "There's nothing we can do about it anyway; things just keep getting worse. Less staff, less funding...And doctors are in charge of everything anyway, and it's not like they ever want anything to change..."

So I say, "I'm really optimistic about the future of health care. Everywhere I go, right across the country, and even in the States and the UK, people are saying they know things can't go on like this. And Canadians really value our health care system. There's a mass consensus that we're not actually going to let anyone destroy public health care. I've also been totally inspired by the young med students. They're not going to tolerate having to work in conditions where people are horrible to one another. I've met so many brave young people who are in med school these days who are willing to stand up and say when things are inappropriate."

Laurie is still barely stifling grimaces and eye rolls, but the rest of the room's mood is lifting slightly. The people who need to go back to work get up and thank me and take cards with my website address, saying that they want to see or read more of the story.

Once they've left, Michelle picks up the discussion again with some very important points about professionals needing to be cognizant of cultural difference when relating to patients.

"So for example, in some Native communities…"

"Yay! Wooo! Native!"

Michelle is interrupted by a nurse named Sara.

When we turn to look at her, she grins. "I'm Native."

Michelle cedes the floor to her. "Please, tell us how this might look different in your community."

Sara looks directly at me, still smiling, and says, "We would all be in there with you the whole time. Our entire community would make decisions with you, we'd smudge you with sweet grass, the whole thing…"

As she mentions the sweet grass, she cups her hands. I can see this so clearly, I can almost smell the burning aromatic fragrance.

Michelle steps in front of me where I'm still sitting on my stretcher and says, "So your community would be there to protect her…" She has her back to me, her arms out-stretched, as if fending off all those who might want to approach me. I breathe it in, feeling my eyes mist slightly. I can imagine this scene with such intensity I feel like it actually just happened. Sara is still smiling at me.

We wrap the room up, and I have an opportunity to chat one-on-one with the participants. I tell Michelle that I think it was really misguided for the Ethics Network to tell me not to talk about politics, and that I think that was what created the challenging moment for the participants, because they felt like I wasn't even remotely acknowledging the conditions they were working in. She looks shocked. "The people at the network told you *what?* That's ridiculous."

"Well, I thought so too. Usually Tommy Douglas shows up."

Michelle leans in with a smile. "I'm the only one reporting back on what you did. It's your story; you take it away and tell it any way you want!"

We make plans to meet shortly before the performance the next day to go over the new material I'm now going to perform. I walk out to the parking lot, where I meet Laurie and she calls me a trailblazer. I tell Laurie that I see this whole situation as just one moment in history. It's easy when we're stuck in the middle of it to start believing that nothing will ever change and that the current state of the world is the way it has always been. But that just isn't true. Any change in our social circumstances has begun as the conscious efforts of groups of people who are dissatisfied with some aspect of the way we're living. Then that very change becomes part of "the way things are"—good or bad. A good example of this is that, prior to the 1940s, people accessed health care through a patchwork of insurance policies through community cooperatives and employers. Because massive unemployment during the Great Depression of the 1930s meant that fewer people were able to pay for doctors' services, a social movement started growing to pressure the government to provide equal access to health care to everyone, regardless of their employment situation. Tommy Douglas was the premier of Saskatchewan at the time, famous for his tenacious attitude and grassroots organizing. He was renowned for his oratory skills and capacity to inspire people through dark moments in history, captured in one of his speeches with the quote, "Courage my friends; 'tis not too late to build a better world." He led a mass movement of men and women, farmers, factory workers, wives, and mothers who were able to pressure the government of Canada to make free access to health care a universal right.

I drive back toward my hotel, stopping at the health food co-op to stock my kitchenette. I'm so relieved. It's always nerve-racking for me to perform previously unperformed material, and this time it was so much worse given the parameters of having to be apolitical. The following morning, I meet up with a close high school friend who now lives in Calgary. Astrid is the chief resident at the hospital where she's qualifying as an anaesthetist. We always have fabulous conversations about patients and doctors—and a good dose of teenaged giggling. It's stuff that none of my other friends would find quite as funny.

Like when my doctor looked at an ulcer above my anus and was really upset because she thought it was a fistula hole burrowing into my bowel. But I'd had this ulcer for about nine years, and it would come and heal and then come back repeatedly. I knew how to treat it using natural salves and cleansers, so I had never even mentioned it to a health care professional. I told the doctor really casually, "Oh, yeah, that's been there forever. It's fine."

And she looked at me gravely and said really slowly, "Julie, you're not supposed to have a hole there."

As if I just lost count of the number of holes in my anatomy. Hilarious. But definitely a story best shared with my medical resident friend Astrid. She invites me to her regular yoga class, where we stretch and enjoy the quiet relaxation.

7. Trail-Blazing Warrior Angels

As I get back into my rental car after hanging out with Astrid, I'm feeling at ease and comfortable, ready to present myself to the awaiting auditorium full of nursing students. Except, when I arrive at the college, the auditorium is empty. There's a cluster of nursing professors sitting at the front, looking a bit fidgety.

"Oh, the students aren't here yet. I'm sure they're still coming."

As I look around the empty two-hundred-seat room, I'm doubtful. It sounds terrible, but honestly, my first thought is, *Meh, whatever. I get paid either way.* We can call it the power of Zen yogic acceptance or just plain indolence, but I happily set up my stage with the knowledge that I might be performing for only eight people.

Michelle and I chat about the previous day in the health care facility. She tells me, "After you left, a bunch of the staff were asking the social worker, 'Why do we never get a chance to talk about these things?' So they've made plans to start an ethics committee where they can regularly have these discussions."

I am thrilled to learn that all the tears in the room resulted in concrete change. The women working in this facility are beginning to demand something different.

We wait another ten minutes. Still no students. The person I start feeling sorry for is the program administrator, who spends a lot of time describing how much work she put into letting the students know. I have no doubt that she did. If you have a situation with only half the students coming, it could mean maybe some people didn't know, but *no one* showing up is clearly about something else.

"Well, they do have mid-terms right now," one professor says.

"They have an essay due in my class," says another.

"My exam is this afternoon," a third prof chimes in.

They're boycotting, I suddenly realize. I look at the professors and remember very clearly the good-heartedness and cluelessness that occasionally accompanies academics in such organizational endeavours. They very honestly believe it's important for their nursing students to witness my patient account of illness and hospitals. And they could have said that there was simply no time to bring me in, because clearly their educational schedule is jam-packed. But adding a voluntary lunchtime event when exams are happening and assignments are due in an environment where students also do hospital practicums is not going to bring out a crowd. The students are clearly overwhelmed and annoyed that their teachers now want them to waste precious study minutes watching some play. If they actually want to prioritize this kind of learning, they need to put it into the curriculum, not as an extra.

There's some generalized eye rolling about "students" and embarrassed glances in my direction. I realize that they think I might be hurt by the low turnout. They couldn't be more wrong. The main thing that is now occurring to me is, *I love teaching the teachers*. If I have an impact on these eight women, it will affect the way they teach all the students anyway. So I go straight into the performance, full force. This time, I hold nothing back. Tommy angelically booms about the disastrous mess his health care system has deteriorated into; I boldly whip out my tampon during the scope scene. The professors get right into it. They love it.

We launch into a very heartfelt and revealing discussion that there's no way on earth these professors would have had in front of their students. We talk about their doubts and fears, moments they still hold that they believe they should have handled differently. Dilemmas in the way they teach.

"What do you recommend for when a student makes a mistake with a patient?" one prof asks me.

"Always tell the truth. Always." I answer quickly and unequivocally. "All they need to say is, 'I'm a student. I'm learning, and I'm going to get someone more experienced now.' And clearly admit to whatever's going on. Then if that patient doesn't want students anymore, the patient has that right."

Michelle, the ethicist, nods. "Clear, informed consent requires honesty."

And I add, "It's also totally possible that the patient will just appreciate the honesty so much that they'll feel safer with the people who admitted to the mistake and not have any issue receiving care from them in the future."

Another prof says, "It's just so hard. We see these types of scenarios going on all the time, where we're all impatient and we don't have time. And we don't want to teach this; we want to change the way nursing students are learning so things will change in the future, but we're really constrained by the lack of resources."

I nod. "For sure, it's a lack of resources that is a major issue. There's also a whole history of medical training that teaches professionals that they're in charge and that, in order to be good doctors, they need to exert power and get unquestioning compliance from patients. I've seen nurses do this too, at the same time as I see how nurses also get disempowered by this set-up."

A nurse who hasn't spoken yet says, "Well, that's why I completely cringed when you talked about your 'angel nurse' during your surgery. Historically we got branded as either these angelic Florence Nightingale figures or as sexpots who provided 'service' to soldiers in wartime. And the doctors were respected and powerful and all-knowing. I'm really tired of the angel archetype; I want nurses to be perceived as strong advocates."

I consider what she's saying, and I think back to why I would describe that nurse who leaned over me during my surgery as an "angel."

I answer carefully. "It's interesting, because I've noticed the angel comes up in a lot of literature when people describe hospital experiences. And for me, it's because in that terrifying crisis moment—where I felt like I could possibly die, and at the very least was undergoing a massive transformation—that nurse was the one who reached out her hand to pull me through to the other side. I also think of angels as warriors. I mean, that's why I describe Tommy Douglas as the archangel of Canadian health care."

"Angel as warrior! I love it." She smiles at me. "Yes, I can see that."

"And patients can be warrior angels too," I point out. "Many people really do want things to change and are absolutely willing to participate in that."

"I used to be a charge nurse in an emerg in Ontario when all the cuts were coming down in the nineties. We had patients lined up in the hallways, just like you described. And I remember patients being really aware of the situation. We had people who were critical right next to the nurses' station and people who were already being treated and stable further down the hall. When new patients came in, the ones next to the station would say, 'I'm feeling better, you can move me down the hall so that they can have my spot.' We had a whole hallway culture thing going on."

It's such a relief to me to think about these moments of collaboration, because health care crises always seem to play out with interpersonal conflicts between patients and professionals or patients and other patients, distracting us all from the reasons *why* we're all scrapping over limited services. I exchange warm goodbyes with the profs and Michelle, the ethicist. They pledge to bring me back and do a better job of getting their students out.

As I'm driving away, I'm taken back to 1996. I was a high school student at the time, and massive protests were happening in downtown Toronto. The entire city was shut down by picketing public service workers and tens of thousands of community supporters. Joanne, our dad, and I wanted to go, so the three of us headed downtown. The legislature lawns were overflowing with flag-waving, picket-sign-toting demonstrators. Blair was somewhere in that crowd too, although we wouldn't meet for another year or so.

The backdrop for these demonstrations was that the federal government in Canada was hell-bent on "balancing the budget." So throughout the 1990s, they slashed billions of dollars from the budgets of the provinces. Just before the 1995 provincial election, Ontario Progressive Conservative Party leader Mike Harris was cooking up a strategy to win the province's top job. He brought in an advisor who'd helped Republican governor Christine Todd Whitman of New Jersey with her "Common Sense Revolution," an idea that Harris wanted to copy. The premise was simple. Blame women who are raising their children in poverty for the economic woes of everyone else. And if someone (like my dad, for example) does have a decent job that allows them to take a family vacation in the summer and pay for kids to get braces, accuse them of being a lazy and useless union worker who's a drain on society. The general "Common Sense" of this approach was to attack people who don't have the resources or social standing to fight and then, while we're all distracted battling it out among our Welfare Queen and Fat Cat Union selves, to funnel massive amounts of our tax money, previously slated for social programs, into providing tax "incentives" for already rich corporations.

So, clearly, you know where I stand on this. But I do have a political science degree, and I also know that reasonable men may reasonably disagree. So I am willing to accept that some people who supported these plans genuinely believed that giving corporations incentives to do business would help the economy and that this newly buoyant economy would ultimately create more wealth for everyone. Some people believed this. Others just wanted special, privatized care for themselves and their rich friends without concern for the good of society as a whole.

These days, I often have this conversation with people at conferences who say, "Health care has enough money; we're just not spending it right." And then conversations with health care professionals whom I'm friends with who say things like, "It's brutal in the emerg. We can't actually give people enough pain medication because we can't afford to put enough staff on at a time to monitor them properly." Whether or not every dollar is spent "right," there is a historical backdrop within the past twenty years that has created the context for the way things are.

So who are the trailblazing warrior angels? They are the ones who came before us, the Tommy Douglases and the thousands of women and men who built the public health care system. They are the angel nurses who hold our hand through surgeries, and the young woman med student who stood up in front of her class to demand justice for a patient. They are the family members who insist on being present when people need them, irrespective of medical protocol. And they are the people advocating right now, rallying with flags and picket signs to demand that their local hospital doesn't get shut down or sold to the highest bidder. Angels are not distant mystical creatures who save us from a terrible world; they are engaged, everyday people who are willing to fight for a better one.

8. Prairie Love

My first prairie performance is in Saskatoon in September 2009.

It's unseasonably warm. Like, thirty-degrees-Celsius warm. The night I arrive, I go to take a voice and yoga class led by a friend of a friend. Later, I walk through some wide open areas where a hot breeze whips up, blowing what feels like desert air, reminiscent of a trip to Tucson six months earlier. It's fall equinox. Time to find some balance.

The following day, I'm performing at a town hall event for a health care conference. The audience is health care professionals, students, and some community members who've come out to make their thoughts about health care known. I'm sharing the stage with an amazing woman called Donna Davis, whom I met the previous spring at another conference. She's a nurse in a very small town in southern Saskatchewan. Several years earlier, she lost her son Vance to medical errors. The inquest following his death blamed "stereotyping" and failing to listen to the family about his condition. When she first told me her story privately, I was outraged by the details. They presumed that, because he was an oil rig worker in his early twenties, his foul mouth was attributable to that. Donna kept insisting that he must have a brain injury because he was an incredibly respectful young man. They ignored her, and he died as a result. Since then, she's become a health care advocate, travelling, telling Vance's story, and becoming a Canadian patient safety representative for the World Health Organization. She's still a nurse in her small town, and in her own work life, she tells me she asks herself every day, "You can be a thundercloud or a rainbow in someone's day—which would you rather be?"

That sums up Donna perfectly. She always chooses the rainbow.

Later at the conference, I meet a young woman who's on her own journey to push change in the health care system. She confides in me that her health issues and subsequent dramas with hospitals and doctors put a massive strain on her marriage.

"That must have happened for you too," she says.

To comfort her, I'd like to answer *yes*. But I can't.

"No, it really didn't. We found this whole new level of closeness and intimacy. Blair felt that this was something that was happening to both of us, not just to me."

Predictably, she looks uncomfortable, and I can practically see her descending into all manner of self-judgment. As I watch this, I realize that although I'm not lying, I'm also not sharing the whole truth. So I clarify.

"It was my recovery that caused the real crisis in our relationship. We needed to find a new way to connect, and it was hard. When we had a common enemy and common goal, we worked together really well. There were things about it that were really nice. I was home so much. I was always present in the relationship. There were concrete things I needed that Blair could provide, and I was always there to listen to him and give him emotional support. When I got well, I was so happy to be feeling good in my body, to have the freedom to go where I wanted when I wanted...that's when the relationship issues really happened."

I don't tell her any more than that. I'm not going to here either, except to say that transitions are always challenging, not just from being healthy to being ill, but from being sick to being well again too.

I'm often approached by young women whose relationships broke down during their illness. As heart-scalding as this is, I always wonder how much longer they really would have wanted to be in that relationship even if they'd never been ill. Life is messy: people get sick, they die, lose jobs, have babies who cry all night, and kids who drive them to distraction—they go bankrupt, have accidents, fail at school, and experience oppression from a world that can't accommodate them. That's just a quick list from people I know well. All of these things either strain our immediate relationships or they teach us to fight together in a brand new way—to take each other's side when it feels like the world is against us.

Everyone falls in love with Blair when they see my show—as well they should; he's fantastic. At the same time, I was never a passive recipient of his love or care. Blair didn't stay with me because he's a selfless martyr, just like I didn't cling to him like a helpless victim. We both chose each other, not because either of us is perfect or because in thirteen years we haven't driven each other completely up the wall at times, but because we *want* to be partners. We chose the relationship—through this and other hard times—because there's so much in it for both of us. Of course, there were times when Blair took care of me physically, nursing me through my illness in ways that I was too ill to return. But no matter how sick I got, I always took care of his heart.

In addition, I was still funny. No matter how bleak things got, we always managed to laugh.

I also don't think that just because I share a common illness experience with people, it necessarily gives us any basis of commonality with regard to our relationships. I had an amazing support system, and I am incredibly grateful to all the people in my life who were with me through my illness. But I'm equally grateful to them for being part of my world right now. Just like when things go on in their lives, exciting or devastating, I'm there for them too. And I was during my illness as well; friends still called with their issues. We still laughed and cried about their stuff as well as mine. I didn't disappear or change or isolate myself in ways that alienated my core group of friends and family. So, as much as I'm grateful, I'm also confident that I was always an equal participant in all of my relationships.

I asked my mother recently what her experience was of me being ill. She said, "I know this word is overused, but you were just so stoic. I never felt like you were needy, like you were desperate or a victim about anything. You just went forward and did everything you needed to do."

I cried when my mum told me this, because I still do feel guilty about how hard my illness was on Blair, my family, and my friends. And that's certainly not my prescription to anyone else of how to behave through illness. Stoicism is highly overrated. I definitely didn't feel that way all the time. I *felt* like I needed them so much. If Blair and my mum were driving to the hospital together, I would lie in fear, imagining how incredibly helpless and alone I would be if their car crashed. I guess I never admitted any of this at the time.

Maia and Dawn shared similar feelings to my mum about their experience of our relationship when I was sick. For them, I was still the same stable, solid me I ever was. My life is always presenting me with new opportunities to become more self-aware and to take responsibility for who I'm becoming and who I want to grow with. I'm forever grateful that Blair, my family, friends, and I all chose to come out on the other side together.

In the following weeks, I travel to three more prairie cities to perform. One of them is Weyburn, Saskatchewan. The conference is for a health region that spans the entire south of the province. The community hall where it's happening is packed. It's a cold prairie day, gearing up to the first snow of the season at nightfall. And the heating is broken in the auditorium. Barefoot in my hospital gown, I feel like my feet are going to fall off as I walk on the frozen stage floor. But the amazing warmth of the crowd quickly thaws me out. They're my favourite type of audience, openly laughing, crying, cringing, and groaning at all the right moments. When I channel the spirit of Tommy Douglas, they start whooping and hollering. I'm having so much fun performing for them I never want to stop. When I finish, they're all on their feet, cheering and clapping. It's my first standing ovation from health care professionals, and I'm overwhelmed. As the emcee returns to the stage to thank me and give me a gift, she asks, "You know this is Tommy Douglas's hometown, right?"

I laugh. "No! I had no idea. I know he was from Saskatchewan, but didn't know where."

I spend the day watching the other speakers and having lots of great conversations with participants. One woman stops me in the kitchen. She's a nurse. She wants to tell me about a patient of hers, a young woman in her early twenties, who died while taking an immune drug for Crohn's disease. I ask her which medication it was, and it turns out to be the one I resisted for so long that I was practically forced into taking. And it's funny because that's not why she approached me. I didn't perform any scenes about that drug. She just wants to connect, to share her own heartbreak at the loss of a patient.

"I still phone her parents," she tells me. "Once a year around the anniversary, just to see how they are, and to see if they want to talk."

Small-town medicine in the prairie tradition of Tommy Douglas is a beautiful thing.

After the conference, a pharmacist who participated is driving me back to my hotel in Regina. I ask him to show me any historical sites around the town related to Tommy. He points directly across the street from the conference building. "Well, that's his church where he was minister." We drive around the block. "And that was his house." As we drive out of town, he takes the route where the giant statue of Tommy greets people on the way in (we'd taken a different road in that morning). I turn to look, and there he stands, seeing us off.

9. Big Bang

Just recently, I emailed my friend Mali, my Vancouver *Buffy*-and-politics co-conspirator, asking her what she wants her pseudonym to be when she appears in the early chapters. She got an academic position down in the States around the time I left Vancouver in 2002, and we've only been in touch on and off since then. We chat back and forth about what we're up to these days and the books we're reading. Over the day and half that we're emailing each other, she gets a message from her family in India. There's a young man, a close family friend, who's been hospitalized in Toronto for Crohn's surgery. He's all alone, and they want to know if she knows anyone who can visit him. When she passes the request on, she says she knows I'm busy, and there's absolutely no pressure, but if I could drop in and see him it would be wonderful.

I notice that I have two reactions as I get this request. The first is that I actually *want* to do it. In the early years of my illness and recovery, such a request would have made me want to hide under a rock. I'd find it almost impossible to say no, even though I'd be horrified at the prospect of visiting the site of someone else's trauma while mine was still so fresh. At the same time, I feel trepidation about the fact that it's a *family* request from continents away, and maybe this young guy doesn't want a strange woman walking into the pain and intimacy of his hospital room.

Mali sends me the details, and I drive to the hospital to see him. He has a very long Indian name that for the purposes of anonymity and ease I'm going to change to Sam. There isn't really a suitable English pseudonym. In these situations, I always feel it's my responsibility to have the basic syllables in someone's name memorized, and I only need to ask once to get the pronunciation perfect from then on.

When I walk into the hospital room, I see a form lying in the bed with sheets pulled so high up on his face that all I can see is a pair of terrified eyes.

I forget entirely what any part of his name is and just stammer uncomfortably. "Hi, um, I'm Mali's friend. Your parents asked if she knew anyone who could come and see you. I'm Julie. I hope you don't mind me coming by."

"Oh, not at all," he says. "It's very nice of you."

"How are you doing?" I ask, the aged and tired question.

"Not too good, actually."

As he tells me about the horror of his last week, he pulls the sheet down far enough that his lips are visible. His story begins on New Year's Eve. He came to Toronto from the town where he's doing his PhD in physics, a couple of hours away. He's at the Greyhound station waiting to get on a bus to New York when he has a bowel bleed so severe that he gets rushed to emergency. They scope him and immediately get him into surgery. That was a week ago. Since then, his blood counts have continued to drop so severely that he's needed multiple blood transfusions. He's still in so much pain at the surgical site that they're going to take a sample to see if there's an infection. He feels dismissed and ignored by swarms of health care professionals marching in and out. He hasn't had the same doctor more than twice.

I sympathize and tell him some of my story, my diagnosis, the periods of medical uncertainty. He looks at me sitting in front of him, well, happy, active, and asks incredulously, "It's possible to recover from this?"

"Yes," I tell him. "It is. Your body is tired and needs some time to repair itself."

Over the course of the past week, no one has told him that he can recover. They come in and out, showering him with medical terminology and clinical tests, but not one single person has told him that his body can heal. The doctors don't understand why his blood count is dropping or why he's still in so much pain. I tell him that in my experience, health care professionals almost always underestimate the trauma of surgery and how long it takes to recover. I tell him his body is just working really hard to recover and his brain just needs to leave it alone to do its job. And I tell him that, as a scientist, he must know that, for everything that is *known*, there's an infinite sea waiting to be discovered—that our grip on the truth is partial at best.

He nods emphatically, agreeing.

"So on some level," I say, "we have no idea why bodies break down when they do or how they miraculously repair themselves."

I tell him the story from 2004, when I was at home lying under my sheet in the throes of yet another medical crisis, feeling like it would never end, and Blair phoned my therapist and passed me the phone under the covers. I will never forget what she said to me: "One day you'll look back at this and you'll think about how brave and strong you were to get through it. You will get to the other side of this. You will do everything you want to do. And right now you just need to rest and take care of yourself." She told me to read novels and watch TV and do whatever I could to just get my mind off of things. Now in 2010, I encourage Sam to watch really bad TV. I point to the small TV attached by an alien-like arm to the corner behind his bed.

"Is your TV hooked up?"

"That's a TV?" He's amazed. "I thought it was just another monitoring device."

I can't believe he's been there for a week and not only has no one told him he can recover from his illness, but no one has told him he has a TV. "I'll go and sort it out and get them to set it up," I tell him.

"Does it cost money?" he asks. "I don't have a credit card."

I wave my hand, "Don't even worry about it. Do you know how many people did things like this for me when I was sick?"

"I'll pay you back as soon as I get out," he says.

"No, no, pay it forward. When you find someone in this situation when you're well and happy and on your feet again, you can do this for them. Seriously, it's my pleasure."

Sam is sitting up farther in his bed now and is talkative to the point of being argumentative. He smiles broadly. "Julie, do you know how small the probability is that I will encounter someone in the exact same situation?"

I laugh. "Sometime something will happen, and in the moment, you'll just know that it's your turn."

I make him promise to watch things that are funny and frivolous. I can tell in most of his life he's very studious and serious, so it takes some insistence before he finally admits to me which sitcoms he likes.

"Well, my friends and I really like *The Big Bang Theory*."

"I love that show!" I tell him. I think about him and his friends doing their physics PhDs, and the recently graduated physicists that Dawn, Blair, and I find so hilarious on the show.

"Are you guys like that?" I ask him.

He laughs loudly and nods.

I leave and sort out the TV. When I return, Sam is sitting up, and his entire body and face is visibly relaxed. I give him my card, a new notebook I've just bought, and a pen, in case he wants to write things down. He says repeatedly, "You're just so kind. You don't even know me."

I don't tell him this, but I do. I *know* him. I know his terror. I know exactly what it is to be alone and to have your disintegrating body being poked by sharp metal instruments and to be dismissed by the white-coated bodies that shuffle in and out. I say goodbye and remind him to email or call, to let me know how it all works out.

The last time I was here in this particular hospital, I visited my Uncle Tony when he had surgery a decade earlier. It was several years before his heart attacks and death.

When I arrived, he was standing in his doorway, IV poles in hand.

"Hi!" he greeted me happily. "I'm just going out for a smoke. Come with me."

So we went down to the concrete patio overhanging a busy downtown street and sat on a bench. He smoked, and we talked about things he was writing and about what I was working on in school. We laughed and joked about our mutual inability to perform well when bosses or teachers are trying to control us. We sat there for almost two hours before he went back to his room and I went to find Blair, who was happily sitting in a café nearby drinking coffee and working on one of his own projects.

Now, ten years later, when I leave this hospital after visiting Sam, I find myself outside the hospital doors in the spot where Uncle Tony and I sat chatting. I linger there for a few minutes and watch the cigarette smoke from other patients wafting by. I like to think that one of the smoke rings is my uncle's — exhaling after a long and satisfying drag from the best cigarette he's ever had. That wherever he is and whatever he's doing right now, he dropped in for a quick, smiling "Hello."

My reverie is interrupted by a loud bang coming from somewhere in the busy downtown street. I rush to the railings at the edge of the concrete landing. A giant dust cloud is obscuring the street from view. People are scrambling in all directions. Gradually, a clearing emerges. Standing in the middle of the street are Frida and Tommy. They're smiling and waving. I feel a hand on my shoulder. I turn — Tony is at my side. They're speaking with one voice, "Julie, it's time," Frida-Tommy-Tony says.

10. Time

I see the three of them together, and I start to cry. It's as if everything I've stored in my body and heart for so long is finally being released. My body is calm, steady, strong. I am breathing deeply as rivers of tears flow easily from my eyes. I'm grinning back at them, understanding without having any words to respond. So I just nod. *It is time.*

Tony joins them in the street. They look so real, so present and solid. They're laughing, and confidence is shining out of them. They link arms and start walking away. I see legions of patients joining them in the street, spilling out into the sidewalk. There's a festival-type atmosphere — equal parts celebration and determination. The wisdom of our bodies, the power of our collective voice inspires great joy. At the same time, it's so clear — we are the bodies that fill the beds, the vessels of disease and health — we need to be the ones guiding health care decisions, from policy to training to the minute-to-minute interactions we have with professionals.

I hold tightly onto the railing with one hand as I enthusiastically wave them off with the other — infused with the energy of the magical march.

That night I start getting emails from Sam's family in India. First from an uncle, then from his mother, then maybe from his father and another uncle — I lose track of who's who. They're thanking me for saving his life. Apparently, Sam described me to them as "an angel." After all the angels who pulled me through, it's amazing to get to play at being one for a little while. But just like none of them saved *my* life, I didn't save his. The greatest gift anyone has given me is to just meet me exactly where I am and support me in making an incremental shift onto more solid ground. And that's all I did for Sam. I didn't give him diet sheets about gluten and dairy. I didn't lecture him about the impact of stress. I mocked the people who were disrespecting him until he laughed so hard he had to take the sheet off his mouth, and told him that his body was strong, that he was getting through this.

I phone Sam a few days later. It's Saturday now.

"Oh, hi," he exclaims enthusiastically when I tell him it's me.

"How are you doing?"

"I'm going home on Monday! My blood work's been fine and they took a sample from my surgical site to see if I had an infection and all the tests came back normal."

"That's great!"

"I'm still in a lot of pain."

"Yeah, for sure. I know. Recovering from surgery can be brutal. But it'll be great to get back to the university and in your apartment with your friends. Do you have people to take care of you?"

"Oh, yes, my friends will."

"And what about school, are they accommodating you?"

"Yes, yes, my supervisor phoned me here and said not to worry about anything, just to take as long as I need to get better."

"That's wonderful. Well, you take care, and stay in touch."

"Yes, and thank you for everything."

"You're *so* welcome."

II. Writing the Ending

I still have a medically contested diagnosis. And by that, I mean that after that dreadful scope, Dr. Gold is still insistent that I have ulcerative colitis, and Athena is sure it's Crohn's. I personally don't care anymore, but seeing as I like her better and Crohn's is easier to say, I alternate between saying "I have colitis" or "I have Crohn's," depending. No diagnosis fully explains the experience and trajectory of an illness, what it's like to *be* a leaky body, day in, day out. But maybe that's the point. Maybe it shouldn't be so easy to pin definitive words with unshaking certainty on these leaky, strong, vulnerable, and beautiful human forms we all walk around in.

All this talk of bodies as battlegrounds is true. We fight so hard to defend this terrain, to martial the boundaries, to resist imposition and encroachment, that sometimes we forget that our bodies are playgrounds too. We stake out our ground with these bodies, these sacred pieces of earth that we live and play in, with such resolve that sometimes we forget to live and play in them. My body is no longer a battleground because I refuse to let it be. I engage the health care system, and the world for that matter, on my own terms.

So these days my life looks more like this—sleep through Blair's alarm and wake up a few hours later. Run a hot Epsom salt bath while I go to the kitchen and make myself a herbal tea and pour a large glass of water. Gradually, I integrate into the waking world, soaking in the bath, sipping tea, and drinking water. Depending on what else I have planned in the day, I might eat and then get dressed and go out to facilitate a writing group, perform a show, give a health care workshop, or go to a meeting at a hospital to discuss patient advocacy. On days like today, I don't get dressed at all. After breakfast, I go back to bed — this time with my laptop, music, tea, and a printed version of this mammoth book. I spend some time procrastinating on the Internet, and then delve deeply back into the pain, terror, and disgust of my twenties because, more recently, the horror of publishing my exposed, raw wounds surfaces. Writing this book is like performing surgery on myself, without gloves or anaesthetic.

And I feel this tension between functionality and authenticity. It's just not practical to walk around with my gashes and inner injuries flapping open and bleeding all the time. Sometimes, I need to paper over the cracks and shore up the leaks just to interact in the world. I can't be a gooey mess all the time. But I can't completely ignore them either, or they just come spilling and raging through on their own terms (generally speaking, out of my bum). So I need to sit with myself and remember that all the yucky difficult crap that comes with being in the world passes. *Everything* passes. And even when I'm sitting in the middle of it, watching it pool around me, multiplying in volume at a seemingly unstoppable rate, and it seems like that's all there is, I remind myself that there's more. This moat of shit will stream away, like every other that has come before it. Flowers will bloom from the extra-fertilized soil beneath, the sun will shine, and all the growth, beauty and joy of being here — being alive and being connected to other people, creating, sharing, and expressing — will explode from my pores with the same intensity as the vileness that kept me stuck here.

Catching colds is a wonderful thing now. I appreciate and find comfort in my immune system's capacity to bring me back to wellness in predictable ways. Day one: sore throat; Day two: headache, fever, runny nose; Night two: soak through the sheets in sweat; Day three: phlegmy cough; and Day four: relief. It's so predictable, comforting, and transient. Efficient.

I'm sitting in my sister's apartment in New York City writing this ending before I finish writing all the chapters in between. I just went and met my friend Kara from high school, who lives in Brooklyn now. We had tapas and drinks and caught up on each other's lives. As I was getting ready to hail a cab, she said, "You know I never really expect the things you're going to tell me, but I also don't *expect* to know what's coming. When I think *Jules*, I think about the way you've always wanted to experience the world. You'd never be satisfied just reading twelve paragraphs about something, you want to dig your hands right into it, whatever it is — to write your own life."

To write my own life. What a beautiful phrasing. When Kara said this, I caught my reflection grinning into her mirrored sunglasses. It was a super-nerdy grin. And although I fixated for several seconds on the combination of my tan making my teeth super-white and the curve of her sunglasses making me look like I had a giant overbite, I quickly returned to the words, and their meaning. I'm not content to have my life written for me; I never have been. I love sitting in this apartment, hearing the street noise below. The beeps, the buzz, the possibility of movement and change. This type of energy and excitement is better for my bowels than any medication. When I feel satisfied that my work is meaningful, when I feel freedom and openness in my life, my digestion is fabulous. My passionate support of people advocating for their own working conditions isn't some principled ethical abstraction. It's a concrete belief that I experience in my own body: creatively participating in the world in ways that are meaningful is healthier for everyone. I do believe in human nature, its compassion and connectedness. The desire to belong, to trust and to be trusted. How can we trust anyone in a world where there are so many barriers to taking care of ourselves and each other?

I find that I still fall brutally and unexpectedly. I come to with my face smooshed into the gravel below. I also find that I get up more easily, confidently, peacefully, gracefully, with less drama. I tend to peek at the endings of books, sometimes before I start reading them, sometimes partway through. It's only fitting then that I should write this ending partway through writing the rest. So this one's for all the peekers. It's a habit I respect. I peek so I can concentrate on the rest of the book without being anxious and perseverating on whether everyone's going to turn out alright. Here's the answer: we all turn out alright, even you. We all made it to this page, a little more bruised and scarred than we were at the beginning, but a lot stronger, and a lot happier too. There were some casualties along the way, but there's a sea of new people that have come to see us through, to march and dance and walk and roll with us, on to the next stages of this journey.

Now we're up north in the woods of snowy Ontario — me, Blair, our dog, Gracie, and our two cats, Willow and Saffy. There's no road access to the cottage, so we have to hike in. There's no hot water, and the plumbing's sketchy, so it's safer to toilet outside in the snow. Earlier today, we took Gracie out for a walk, and I noticed a feeling of lightness as we left. I wasn't carrying a bag, and Gracie's fine off-leash up here, so I thought that explained the feeling. I considered it a bit more and realized that I didn't feel lighter compared to walking in our neighbourhood in the city; I felt lighter in my body. I walked away from the building with no anxiety about pain and being far from home if I suddenly needed the washroom. This fear, which I used to carry as a constant, back-breaking load, is gone. It happened so gradually I almost didn't notice it leaving, until here I am, free in my own body.

Acknowledgements

The excerpt from "Variations on the Word Sleep" by Margaret Atwood is from *True Stories*, copyright 1981. Published by Oxford University Press and reprinted by permission.

I often discuss writing with my dear friend Lorraine Hussey. We always conclude that every essay, article, and book is the product of a thousand conversations. In every one of these conversations, we stand on the shoulders of millions of people who have advanced thought through experience, discussion, and reading hundreds of other people's work. Writers, as such, are labourers. We are the storytellers of our communities who do our best to express the thoughts and feelings we have developed through our relationships with others. As such, I owe acknowledgement to more people than I can possibly name here. Any insight that you find useful or moving in these pages was drawn through extensive discussion with the brilliant people I have been lucky enough to share space with in the last ten years. Anything that makes you cringe is entirely my fault. That said, I offer tremendous gratitude to this very incomplete list of people.

Natalie Atkinson, for her huge, open heart and for understanding me like no one else. Lorraine Hussey, for her brilliance and impassioned support. Michelle

Robidoux, for political wisdom and steadfastness through so many things. Dave Molenhuis, whose friendship and creative collaboration were instrumental in finishing this book.

My three goddesses of theatre: first, my amazingly talented soul sister and director Suzanne Roberts-Smith, for bringing her fire to my work; Creative Facilitator extraordinaire Katherine Duncanson, for bringing so much joy; and Margot Massie, for everything theatrical and otherwise—your imprint is still on these pages.

The three wise men who navigated the world of publishing with me: fellow writer Micah Toub, who talked me down from many literary cliffs and self-defeating positions; editor Jonathan Schmidt, for his unparalleled enthusiasm from the beginning and for making space for Frida Kahlo and Tommy Douglas to burst out into text; and finally, my agent Chris Bucci, for his sage advice, patience, and commitment to getting this book published. And everyone else at the Anne McDermid Agency, who also stood by this project and defended it in rough literary times, especially Martha Magor, who was present and supportive in some crucial moments.

Susanne Alexander, Colleen Kitts, Corey Redekop, James Duplacey, Chris Tompkins, and all the staff at Goose Lane Editions—thank you, thank you, thank you—me and my leaky body will be forever grateful that you brought this story to the page. And also Heather Sangster from Strong Finish (who I would now like to copy-edit my life).

Heather Mallick, Diane Flacks, and Brian Goldman, for an incredibly supportive introduction of my leaky body to the wild world of media.

The Ontario Arts Council Writers' Reserve, for financial support in 2009—and to everyone at the various publishers who read, sent notes, and recommended funding, especially Amanda Crocker at Between the Lines, who has been incredibly supportive throughout.

Margrit Shildrick, author of *Leaky Bodies and Boundaries: Feminism, Postmodernism and (Bio)ethics,* for her generous theoretical insights and for shaping my understanding of bodies, medicine, performance, and experience. Marcia Rioux, Valorie Crooks, Geoffrey Reaume, and everyone at the Critical Disability Studies graduate program at York University for academic guidance and inspiration throughout. Diane Driedger and Michelle Owen, for publishing versions of this story in anthologies, and to the *Canadian Theatre Review,* for showcasing my work in Spring 2011. And in the beginning, high school English and Drama teachers Sarah Holding and Paul Murray, who assured me this was all possible decades ago.

Julie Righter and Tony Greco, for emotional and psychological support during the ill years, and Sandra Moon Dancer and Diana Griffin, for spiritual and physical support during the healing years — I honestly don't know how I would have survived without you. Infinite gratitude to Moon Dancer in particular, who saw health where I saw disease and envisioned possibilities where I saw dead ends.

Patients, health care professionals, and loved ones, who after shows, in workshops, and in hundreds of emails have shared incredible vulnerability and insights that have guided me through. Gilda's Club in Toronto has been a wonderful venue for these conversations; much thanks to Maureen Aslin for making me so welcome there.

The staff at The One and Only Coffee house, for keeping me in almond milk lattes and politely looking away as I quietly wept in corners while writing and doing edits.

Kelly Holloway, Kim Persaud, and Jesse McLaren, for their honest feedback on the first draft in 2004 and advice in the early stages—your voices have been in my head these last eight years as I have written, revised, and re-written.

Through the years it has been my great privilege to call the following people my friends—Meg and Rosie Fenwick, Lorraine Chow, Sandra Ferreira, Kevin Tonon, Bradley Hughes, Brynn Bourke, Kim Walker, Charlotte Ireland, Linda Muraca, Christine Beckermann, Jenna Simpson, Serena Oakley, Samantha Lowes, Chantal Sundaram, Jordana Greenblatt, Jijian Voronka, Samantha George, Tithi Bhattacharya, and Fania Beviil—it would require a whole other book to describe how important you've all been in this process.

My parents, Lucia and Kevin, my sister Joanne, my Aunty Mary, for being a wonderful family and especially for your remarkable faith in my writing. And to my in-laws, Bernice and Albert. There was never a time I felt anything other than complete support from all of you in this project. Much love.

Finally to Blair—my life partner and soulmate. I love you times twelve billion. Plus infinity. Plus one.

Notes

I would like to acknowledge the sources of the following material.

Epigraph. Taken from the tombstone of Tommy Douglas, Beechwood Cemetery, Ottawa, Ontario.

p. 86. Excerpt from *The Wizard of Oz* screenplay by Noel Langley, Florence Ryerson, and Edgar Allen Woolf. Based on the book by L. Frank Baum (Metro-Goldwyn-Mayer, 1939).

p. 137. Excerpt from *Wit* by Margaret Edson (New York: Dramatists Play Service, Inc., 1999).

P. 217. Excerpt from *Fall on Your Knees* by Ann-Marie MacDonald (Toronto: Vintage Canada, 1997).

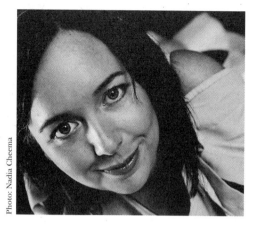

Julie Devaney is a patient-expert in the fields of disability rights advocacy and health care delivery. She is the writer of the critically acclaimed show and educational workshop series *My Leaky Body,* which she has performed at medical schools, nursing conferences, disability and women's studies conferences, arts festivals, and theatres throughout Canada and in the US and the UK, including a successful run at Theatre Passe Muraille in Toronto.

Devaney was named a Woman Health Hero by *Best Health Magazine* in 2011 and has been profiled on CBC Radio's *White Coat, Black Art,* and in *Chatelaine, Abilities Magazine,* and the *Toronto Star.* Her writing has appeared in *The Huffington Post, The Globe and Mail,* and in numerous anthologies.